Yoga for Age 60+

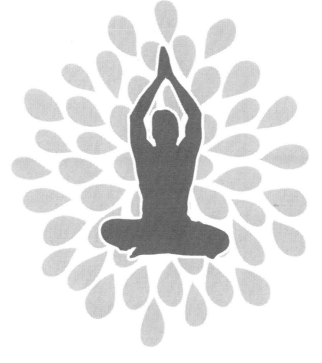

A Guide to a New Journey
of Safe Yoga Practice at Home

By Meena Vad

Illustrations by George Matchen

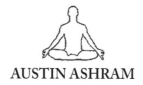

AUSTIN ASHRAM

ISBN-10: 0984532420
ISBN-13: 978-0984532421
Library of Congress Control Number: 2011914160

For more information, or to order additional copies, please contact:

Austin Ashram
5501-A Balcones Dr. Ste. #207
Austin, TX 78731
USA
+1 (512) 786-7931

www.Austinashram.com/yogafor60
Quantity discounts available.

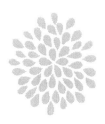

I would like to dedicate this book to all who practice Yoga and to those who will decide to start this practice!

Contents

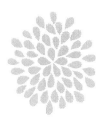

Acknowledgments

I would like to express my gratitude and love to the following people:

To all my Yoga teachers, the knowledge of Yoga that you have given me is a real treasure of infinite value.

To my dear friends and family members, for sharing of your experience of Yoga practice, and giving me amazing insights. Your input for this book is tremendously valuable.

To my son Vik, your inspiration, encouragement and support made this book possible.

To my daughter Chanda, for time spent in editing the manuscript. Your input and suggestions are a big help to me.

To George, thanks for providing accurate Yoga illustrations.

To Austin Ashram, many thanks for your support and help in this endeavor.

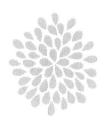

Preface

Thoughts about the mystery of life are always on our mind but the ones that come to mind more often at the age of sixty and after, are "How long will I live?"; "What will be the quality of my life?"; "How am I aging?"; and "I want to live in good health for the rest of my life but is there a way to have good health later in life?" The answer to the last question is yes; there is a way to live in good health without worrying about aging and we can experience it when we practice Yoga. This answer comes from the ancient scientists and from modern scientists who have conducted numerous studies to determine the results of Yoga practice.

Talking to my friends and family members about their Yoga practice and their experiences with it gave me some insights and a better understanding of Yoga. Their actual stories about the benefits they had received inspired me to write this book. I saw the effects of Yoga practice on people when I was a child, and I became interested in finding out more about it. My personal experience with Yoga was a great help during my working years and when raising my children. When I was facing some health problems in my forties and fifties, the regular practice of Yoga strengthened me, so I would like to share with my readers this new way toward their well-being and fitness beyond age sixty.

I have put this information together as a practitioner of Yoga and as a researcher, gathering this information for the last fifty years. The possibilities of good health and well-being that Yoga provides are available to all, no matter what condition your body and mind are in.

Scientific research shows that Yoga makes a difference toward enhancing our strength of body and mind beyond age sixty and for the rest of our lives. This is a guide to wellness beyond age sixty and a step-by-step approach to the safe practice of Yoga.

This book will give you all the information you need to start your safe Yoga practice at home. There is no place like home to practice Yoga. The comfort of your home and the familiarity of your surroundings make you relax easily. I suggest that you read the entire book first. The first and second chapter describe your life so far, your life after sixty, and the possibilities of good health with Yoga practice. Chapters 3 and 4 describe Yoga, its origin, the types of Yoga, and how to prepare for Yoga practice at home. Chapters 5 and 6 will give you detailed information about the steps you need for Yoga postures. Chapters 7, 8, and 9 describe the Yoga of Breathing, Meditation, and Devotion. Chapter 10 alphabetically lists specific health conditions and describes postures that will be helpful for these conditions. The last two chapters, 11 and 12, provide some guidance toward healthy life choices. The techniques that are described here are for prevention and maintenance of good health and are only for educational purposes. They should not be used to treat or diagnose a disorder. You are the best judge to choose which Yoga exercises suit you. You will find that spending a small amount of time doing Yoga can create such a meaningful improvement in your life. As you start your Yoga practice, I wish you more strength, flexibility, peace of mind, and good health!

Meena Vad

1 Your life so far

Life is a series of choices!

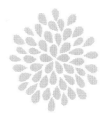

Go ahead and look in the mirror!

Who do you see? You are looking at a being with a vast amount of data stored in your memory. Your life experience so far can be considered your "gathering and storage" of a large amount of data. Your beliefs, growing-up experiences, your working life, family life, your experiences in dealing with difficulties and managing your life—all your experiences together—have created this data. You have become a supercomputer with a huge memory and a large amount of data storage. Each person is a unique supercomputer because each person has unique experiences and unique perspectives. This data includes your abilities and skills, your successes and failures, your triumphs and tragedies, your gains and losses, all the events you participated in, all the people in your life, and what you gave and received. You have traveled a long way! And along this way, you have experienced the whole spectrum of emotions, from joy to sorrow, and from pleasure to pain. Also along the way, you have gained some knowledge. This knowledge is yours to keep.

This journey so far shows us how we have evolved. This process of evolution and data storage continues all our life.

We can make this data and our knowledge our treasure and use it for our benefit. Think about the processing that goes on continuously in the brain. We accumulate millions of bits of data every day. This data affects our thinking and our decisions. Yoga practice gives us the ability to digest this data properly, sort and store it effectively, and manage it efficiently so it can be used for our benefit all our life. The previously acquired experiences and information give us the ability to have a quick memory recall and a better understanding, as well as the ability to draw conclusions quickly and to make right decisions. Wisdom and mature perspective are hard-won prizes indeed! The precious memories from the past and the external pleasures will remain with us all our life, but there is more to life.

We see that most people in this sixty-plus age group experience a lack of energy and tiredness, with or without some health problems. The question that comes to mind is should we continue to live like this or change our life for the better? When we decide to change it, we need to think about what Yoga can offer. The focus of Yoga is on keeping the body supple and strong and the mind relaxed, focused, and powerful. Yoga is not competitive, not religious, and you can start the safe practice of Yoga any time, at any age in your life, no matter what condition of health you have.

We all want the ability to function well, have financial security, freedom from diseases, peace of mind, usefulness, happiness, and quality relationships with family and friends. We don't get these automatically; we need to go for them and work for them for the rest of our life. Life is a series of choices; the choices we make go toward the fulfillment of our desires. The greatest desires in life, like food, clothes, money, houses, status, sex, cars, land, and things of pleasure, are achieved by all, to some extent.

After we get these things in life, we think we will be happy. However, in reality, we find that even after we have all these things, we still have fear, doubts, struggles, and conflicts inside us. They did not go away. Seeing this, we get dissatisfied. We want something else; we have an inherent "need" of something deeper. That "something deeper" in us is called our authentic self, or higher self. We want to get in touch with that hidden part of us. Our life is our journey to experience the higher self. We get some glimpses of it when we have a gut feeling or an insight or when we are creative or love without conditions or when we pray deeply.

Our body and mind have brought us where we are today. It was a long journey. It was not easy a lot of times. Now it is time to nurture these two important parts of ourselves. What is needed for us is some internal nurturing, not external nurturing. We did the external nurturing for many years.

We create our sense of self out of remembering our life experiences. In life, most of us have been more focused on "externals"—other people, professions, immediate gratification, and use of external things and means like good food, nice clothes, houses, possessions, trips, sports, and hobbies. We have given importance to what other people think about us rather than what our inner voice says and what our deep beliefs tell us; then we reacted to life in that "external" way. Our parents and teachers expected us to behave in certain ways in childhood. Our friends, spouses, and co-workers expected us to behave in certain ways. We agreed to the ways of society, and that created who we are. Our own will was there, but it was conformed to the structure in which we live and it got mixed with other people's wills. Many times, we ignored the subtle voice we heard from our body or mind, which was trying to show us the beneficial way, but we went ahead with what was required from us. Then a conflicting environment was created within ourselves.

3

This caused difficulties then, and more of the difficulties we see now, in the form of some disorders, pain, depletion of energy, and diseases. We were focused on un-beneficial factors. We were addicted to "doing"; we were involved too much with our "to do" lists every day. Right after we woke up, our agenda for the day would start and go on until we fell asleep at night. The "to do" habit never ended, day after day, month after month, year after year. The lists got modified a little, but would continue on and on. Even when vacationing or relaxing, our mind was busy with our "to do" lists; the thoughts about them would not leave us. Think about how much energy we spent in doing that. Some of it, of course, was needed in order for our life to go on but a lot of it made us tired and even exhausted. No wonder we are restless all the time, even when we sleep. Sleep cannot restore the balance in us and we become susceptible to some health problems, disorders, and diseases. Then we add more to our "to do" lists with health matters. Every human being needs some quiet time each day to check on feelings, needs, wants, and goals; but we tend to fill even our free time with activities. Our body and mind crave deep rest every day, but do not receive it.

Millions of people are finding themselves on the journey of life after sixty and beyond. By the year 2020, one out of every six Americans will be over the age of sixty-five. The same trend is occurring worldwide. The predominant view we see regarding the senior years is that it is equated with weakness, disorders, diseases, and suffering. We know now that growing older does not necessarily mean getting sicker. We see more and more centenarians in the world today who live happy lives. Their good health and positive mental outlook are their secrets.

The question is how much importance are we willing to give to making our later life healthy and productive? We need to make a crucial choice from the depth of our heart to go for it. We have the potential to do it.

We have made some right choices regarding our health and we have made some wrong choices in the past. Sometimes, even though we knew some choices were wrong, we went ahead with them. One of my former co-workers, Ken, blamed himself for smoking for the last forty years. He was having some breathing difficulties. He said, "I try to stop smoking but I feel helpless; my habit is controlling me." I knew that he honestly had tried to stop it with many different methods. He knew the cause and effect relationship. He added, "You know, just knowing about it is not enough. One part of my mind wants to stop it, but the other part and the body doesn't go with it." Ken had to retire early because of his emphysema and breathing problems.

There is hope for Ken; and there is hope for all who suffer from health problems. The recent studies on aging show us that the brain is more capable of self-repair than we think. We need to remember this when we are under the influence of age-related difficulties. We know that our body responds to the way we think, feel, and behave. When we are upset, angry, or are under stress, our body shows it to us by responding with aches and pain, headaches, tiredness, or upset stomachs. If we stay in these states for a long time, we develop serious disorders and diseases. We can use this suffering and pain to serve and guide us toward a better way, toward learning something from it, and modify our ways. In order to get out of our health-related difficulties, we need to shift our focus from the externals to our internals and focus on our body and our mind. These two are the only means that give us good health and well-being.

There is a connection between belief and biology. Our belief system causes us to age. Seeing people around us grow old and feeble and die, we believe that that is the way the life flows. We learn that, for centuries in the past, human beings were exposed to the harsh environment, famines, natural disasters, inadequate nutrition, physical labor, epidemics of diseases, and

5

lack of medical help. It puts a picture in our mind that aging is inevitable, normal, painful, and also fatal. But as we learn the new ways and our external environment gets better, we see that aging is very personal; with a healthy lifestyle, we can eliminate or lessen the symptoms of aging. With positive influences in our external and internal environment, our organs can function in a healthy way.

Aging is not the same in all societies around the world. In the U.S. and Europe, heart disease, cancer, and diabetes are major causes of deterioration of health, and they cause rapid aging. Gerontologists are finding that some societies like Venezuela, Okinawa, the Solomon islands, and in the Mediterranean, people remain active and healthy in later years. They found out that the reasons for their good health were moderate and fresh diets, daily exercise, social bonds, inclusiveness, leisure time, togetherness of young and old, a slower pace of life, giving a helping hand to each other, sharing their feelings, friendships, rituals, and an attitude of contentedness. All these factors contribute to the well-being of the members of these societies, and thus aging is delayed for them. In technologically advanced societies, these factors are lacking. Importance is given to instant gratification, a fast-paced life, unhealthy eating habits, greed for money, and for material things, exclusiveness, and a "me only" way of life.

The age of a person consists of three complex factors:
Chronological age – calendar age
Biological age – age of the body in terms of cellular processes
Psychological age – how old we feel
The chronological age is unchangeable, but biological age and psychological age are changeable and are also personal. It is to our benefit to pay attention to what is changeable and find ways to change for the better. Once we become aware of these factors, we can change our thinking. Awareness has the ability to influence our aging. Life is awareness flowing with action.

The question arises, how do we focus on awareness and on our body and mind? Yoga practice gives us the way to do it. It creates that focus as we practice Yoga. It is a great science and easy to learn. I have seen it work in the last fifty years of my life for all age groups, but especially well for the sixty-plus age group. I have observed the difference between Yoga practitioners and non-practitioners, and was impressed to see what Yoga can do for practitioners in later years. As a researcher and a practitioner of Yoga, I have gathered a lot of data over the years. It clearly shows the amazing benefits of Yoga well into the later years of life.

Take this quiz to see how you are progressing at this stage in life.

No.	Facts	Applies strongly: 10 points	Applies 50% of the time: 5 points	Applies rarely: 2 points	Does not apply: 0 points
1	I spend about 30 minutes in some kind of exercise every day				
2	I do not get upset easily when things don't go according to my plan				

7

No.	Facts	Applies strongly: 10 points	Applies 50% of the time: 5 points	Applies rarely: 2 points	Does not apply: 0 points
3	I eat 3 balanced meals every day				
4	I spend some time with my friends at least once a week.				
5	I spend some time in prayers or some kind of spiritual practice each day				
6	I have tried new things or new hobbies or new pursuits in the last 12 months				
7	I feel comfortable and at peace with myself when I am alone				

No.	Facts	Applies strongly: 10 points	Applies 50% of the time: 5 points	Applies rarely: 2 points	Does not apply: 0 points
8	I do not dwell too much on past events				
9	I sleep five or more hours every night				
10	I do not smoke or use tobacco products				
11	I do not consume alcohol				
12	I focus on the positive aspect in people, situations and events				
13	My relationships with my family and friends is a happy one				
14	I regularly help around the house				

Total points:

A total score between 100 and 140 points – You are healthy and will live for many years. You have flexibility of mind and have good habits. A regular Yoga practice will be useful in helping you maintain your health.

A total score between 40 and 99 points – You can become aware of your habits and then modify them for better health. The regular practice of Yoga will enable you to change some of your patterns of life for the better.

A total score of 39 points and below – Some major changes will enhance your life and your health. Implementing Yoga practice into your routine and continuing with it, will add more energy and better health to your life.

No matter what your score is, Yoga will definitely enhance the quality of your life. It will add more zest, meaning, and joy to your life. As we shift our focus to the "core" of our being, we discover a whole new world! In order to get in touch with our core, what we need is a life strategy for the next part of our life! In the coming chapters, we will see how we can achieve better health and a better life with Yoga practice, and see the best part of our life that is yet to come!

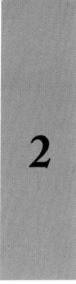

2

The next part of your life

*Yoga practice
makes the future part of your life
better than the present!*

One mystery of life is that we don't know how long we are going to live. Keeping this unknown factor in mind, we want to live in good health with comfort and peace of mind. No matter what our age is, no matter what condition of health we have, Yoga is there for us. It helps our body and mind and makes both stronger and healthier. It gives us inner peace that goes very deep. Since I was a child, I have seen many people who practiced Yoga and have observed that they had something that other people did not. My fascination with Yoga has grown since then; I have been gathering some data on Yoga and people's experience with it. I was fascinated to see the effects of Yoga in later years of life for many people. After seeing the numerous experiences of these people, I noticed a common thread in Yoga-practitioners.

I would like to present it to you as you are thinking about the next part of your life.

We hear that heart disease is the number one killer of both men and women in the United States, that every twenty seconds someone has a heart attack. We face the facts that one person in every four in the sixty-plus age group suffers from diabetes, and stroke risk increases with age. We are concerned when we hear this, but thanks to the years of research and scientific break-throughs, we do not have to accept aging as inevitable. We do not have to feel tiredness and weakness, or suffer from debilitat-ing conditions. We do not have to feel feeble and worn out. We do not have to comply with the thought that sleep gets less and less as you age. We all want to be free from suffering.

As soon as we feel pain in our body, we try to get rid of it as quickly as possible. Most of the time, we use the quick band-aid approach. Sometimes it works, but most of the time it does not. We try medications and we have to deal with their side effects. When we feel anger, fear, stress, or worry, it is painful for the body and mind. If these states are held over a long time, they turn into rage, depression, worthlessness, or a serious disease. Then we add more medications and more side effects on top of the original problems. The root cause of all these problems remains hidden. If we can remove the root cause, we will be much healthier. But how do we find the root cause?

The good news is that no matter what happened in the past, we can move beyond our past limitations. The practice of Yoga offers the connection to the inner workings of our body and mind. As we go deeper in our practice of Yoga, we feel this connection and we see this connection. It gives us a better understanding of our problems. We gain access to the knowledge of the root cause. The next step then is to modify our ways. With the practice of Yoga, it becomes easier to modify our ways.

Actually, the sixty-plus time period can be the most enjoyable time period when we are free from many obligations. We can have new hobbies, we can travel and see new places, learn something new, spend more time with friends, have some meaningful activities, or just relax more at home or be alone and enjoy the peacefulness. The freedom is there, and we need to use it to our benefit. We certainly do not want to spend this time in sickness and pain. We need to be free from our unpleasant past. We can always keep the pleasant memories of our past and cherish them, but letting go of the troubled and unpleasant past is a very important skill. There is no sense in carrying the burdensome past. Yet the past seems to control our behavior and our ways.

The impressions of our past, the decisions we made in the past, the way we faced situations, all come to the surface in every situation now, in the present. If we need to make our life comfortable, we need to change the effects of the past. The stored memories of our past are like grooves in the mind. They send the same messages again and again. This results in a fixed or rigid reaction to situations. An example of this is a controlling person who tries to force other people and events to his/her way of thinking. This behavior arises from insecurity and being afraid of letting others be who they are. Controlling people are always tense and complaining. Other people do not feel comfortable or relaxed in their presence. In order to change this behavior, a controlling person needs to look inside and see the effects of this behavior. Many people avoid looking inside.

My neighbors, an elderly couple, Roger and Alice, are set in their ways. Roger is the decision maker and controller in every aspect of their life. Alice is into complying with everything, but is frustrated. She wants Roger to change his ways, but Roger says, "I'm the way I am; I can't help it." At some level in his mind, he has decided that change is not possible or he is not willing to try to change because a change means giving up control. It means the deep insecure part of his mind is afraid to change. If he sees that fear clearly, he surely will be able to remove it.

Yoga practice gives the ability to get to the deeper levels of the mind. Then we can see clearly how our thoughts affect our behavior and our life. Once we see it, we can reprogram our thoughts for better results.

Now is the time to look into the internal realm. In our prayers, we pay attention to our internal world. Let us go a little deeper into it. We can start it with Yoga practice and begin this new journey. Life is, basically, a journey of consciousness or awareness. We were not aware of many things before, either outside of us or inside of us. As we become aware of our physical, mental, emotional, and spiritual states, we can change for the better and our life becomes better. This journey itself is really fascinating, with a reward of growth and expansion along the way. As we become conscious of our own thought process and underlying belief systems, we can see that there are more thoughts available that might be more beneficial to us. This journey allows us to look into our own inner landscape. In this landscape, we can discard what is not useful and plant what is beneficial to us.

In the mid '80s in my Yoga class, I met Jim and his wife Donna. They both started doing Yoga two years earlier after Jim retired from his work. They wanted to learn more because they saw what Yoga was doing for them. Jim said, "The tiredness and the pain in my lower back is gone now and I have more energy. I thought I was stuck with pain and medications for the rest of my life but you know, I started a wood workshop in my garage two months ago and I teach my students how to make wooden toys." Donna looked relaxed, as her insomnia was disappearing slowly. I told them about my migraine headaches that were getting less as I started a regular practice of Yoga. We all agreed that we need to learn more about Yoga since there is a lot more available. We felt the newness of life every time we shared our Yoga-practice experiences over the years.

Sometimes, with health conditions such as back pain, stiffness, or weight gain that we experience after age sixty, we tend to think that we are stuck with them for the rest of our life. This thought of getting stuck makes us even weaker than the actual condition, and the medications for it give us side effects that are an additional burden to bear. Yoga practice gives us the ability to go past this weakness and gain strength. When our body and mind work together, it can give us good health and well-being for the rest of our life. Yoga practice creates a change in you. It means that the body and mind had the ability to heal all along. It was just that the door was closed. Yoga will open that door so we can have the well-being that we all value so much. We can see the possibility of staying fit and healthy beyond sixty and for the rest of our lives. We need to accept changes in our body as natural changes, not as crises.

There are some disabilities you cannot change. The great inspirational teacher, minister, and author of *The Power of Positive Thinking*, Dr. Norman Vincent Peale said, "The secret of life isn't what happens to you but what you do with what happens to you." Yoga practice gives us the ability to do what is the best for our present condition. It enables us to manage our life effectively so that we remain functional and self-reliant. We want the ability to prevent disorders, manage them well if we have them, and significantly reduce their impact, and to have the strength to endure and improve them if there is no other way. Yoga practice makes this possible. It is like depositing some of your hard-earned money in a savings account in the bank. You feel the peace of having it and it comes in handy when there is a need of it. Along with that, you get a heap of satisfaction and self-confidence.

My first experience with Yoga happened in India when I was eight years old. During summer break, on a bright morning, my father said, "I am going to teach you the Sun Salutations today. Just follow the sequence that I show you; these steps need to be done in a certain order." Being a mathematics professor with an authoritative voice, my two brothers and I couldn't ask our father any questions or protest or say anything. We did as we were told. We were outside on the patio, in the morning sun, and the air was warm. On a large mat, I started the steps of the Yoga exercise of the Sun salutations, facing the Sun. After a few rounds, I got the sequence of twelve poses right. It felt good and I felt a certain lightness in my body. After that lesson, I wanted to practice it every morning. I continued it for a while then stopped it and started again. The starting and stopping went on for years. With my educational background of a degree in physics, I look at the world in a scientific way rather than an emotional one, and also in a more skeptical rather than accepting way. At that time, the dazzle of the scientific breakthroughs and technological innovations were overwhelming. In that flow of modern life, the ancient wisdom of Yoga went on the back burner. But in the 1970s and '80s, a lot of scientific studies on Yoga and meditation were going on in many universities, and they were publishing amazing results from the practice of Yoga. In my late twenties in the U.S., when I started to feel tiredness every day, I went back to it, blaming myself for not practicing for so long. It was helping me a lot. Still, as a working wife and mother, taking care of three children, housework, job stress, and the ups and downs of life, my practice was not so regular. In my forties, I started twice weekly Yoga practice and it helped me with my migraine headaches and feet aches. In my fifties, when I experienced elevated blood pressure, I resolved to practice Yoga on a daily basis. I tried medication for my blood pressure but it didn't help much, so after consulting with my physician, I decided to rely on Yoga practice and meditation without any medication. It is working for me.

What we are seeking is not necessarily the longevity of life but a better quality of life, however long it lasts. The average life expectancy in the world today is sixty-six years, compared with forty-six years only seventy years ago. In the United States, the average life expectancy is seventy-six years. We need to remove the factors that compromise the quality of life, especially in later years. As we focus on improving the quality of our life, what we need is some changes and some flexibility. These changes will get us out of our set patterns; some old habits will be replaced by new ones. Once we are able to handle the changes, the next part of our life will be a lot better.

We know that "change" is our lifelong companion. When we keep our attitude of wonder, curiosity, and joy toward the change, we will remain in the flow of life. Yoga practice actually creates in us the ability to handle changes. What more can you ask for?

As we live a healthier and happier life by practicing Yoga, we have the potential to make important contributions to society in later years. The senior generation is the foundation of any society in any nation. It is our responsibility to keep this foundation strong and stable and not let it get weaker. In the upcoming chapters, we will see how we can achieve this goal.

3 What is Yoga and what can it do for you?

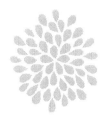

Yoga is a science that originated in India about eight thousand years ago. The great sages used the principles and theories of the mind-body connection, studied them, experimented with them, and then developed the science of Yoga. They perfected it as a practice that anyone can use. Yoga means *unity* or *oneness* and is derived from the Sanskrit word "yuj," which means "to join" or "to unite." Yoga practice enables us to join our body and mind, and we join our energy with the Universal Energy. Yoga is a science, like any other branch of science, and if you follow it correctly, it will definitely give you results. And what are the results? They include good health, energy, flexibility of body and mind, healing from disorders, freedom from pains, balance, expanded intellectual capacity, self-control, better sleep, and rejuvenation. The science of Yoga begins with the outermost aspect of a person, the physical body, and then moves on to mental, intellectual, emotional, and spiritual levels. The principles underlying the ideas in the Yoga scriptures are fresh and dynamic. The science of Yoga proposes to give us the means of observing our internal states of body and mind. The instrument is the mind itself. The most important thing is that these ideas do work and produce results. They stand on their own merit. There is no need to change your way of life; just adding Yoga practice will enhance what you do.

In Yoga practice, the dormant energies in our body and mind get activated. We usually do not use all our capabilities; they lie dormant and remain unused. The intelligence of the cells in our body comes to play an important part in our life. Yoga awakens the body's dormant electro-magnetic energies, gives an internal massage to the heart and to all organs, produces brain-coherence, and strengthens the nervous system. It provides the integration of physical, mental, emotional, and spiritual aspects of us. Yoga practice is the process of polishing the brilliant, shining "Gem of the Self," which got clouded or dusty due to our ignorance. It is the knowing that inside us, we possess something far greater than the material things we possess in the outer world.

In the physical body, various organs and systems have their own function, and there is interrelationship and coordination between them. If any of the system (for example, the digestive system) is in ill health, it affects the rest of the systems. In the same way, if you create balance in one system, the result is a balance in other systems. Yoga helps us to create that balance in our body and mind. During Yoga practice, a natural realignment occurs in the body and it leads to a natural realignment of your perception of life.

The benefits of Yoga go beyond the physical part. After your Yoga practice, you will feel centered and calm, and you can stay focused. Many people say that after their Yoga practice, their thoughts are positive and happy. Yoga practice changes the state of the body and mind by infusing some kind of energy. You get a new ability to deal with life's challenges. It helps you in your everyday life, in your work, in your leisure, in your relationships, and in your role as a useful member of society, regardless of your age. Doing Yoga practice daily is the key to gaining strength and flexibility. It is a process of reenergizing yourself. Once you feel it, you want to reenergize yourself daily.

Yoga opens the path toward the "core" of you. That core is the most powerful part of you. You would want to be connected to it. Why? It's because the power flows from there. You can use this power in all areas of your life. Today, Yoga is practiced in all countries by people from all religions. Yoga is not attached to any particular religion. It is a way of healthy life. Yoga advocates proper eating habits, but you do not have to be a vegetarian to practice Yoga. Yoga is not just physical exercise, not something you read, know, and understand, or talk and discuss, it is something you practice to experience the power within you. It is a firsthand personal experience that you feel inside yourself.

Yoga has been accepted as a therapeutic science all over the world, and many scientific studies have been conducted. Yoga is gaining respect among doctors and medical researchers. There has been an explosion of data using Yoga as a treatment option. Numerous studies at many universities in several countries have found that Yoga helps people suffering from hypertension, anxiety, depression, arthritis, stress, diabetes, epilepsy, cancer, weight problems, and many disorders. These are the current scientific verifications of what the great sages told us a long, long time ago. The studies done by the National Institute of Health (NIH) and National Center for Complementary and Alternative Medicine (NCCAM) suggest that real benefits are obtained through consistent and regular practice of Yoga. Clinical studies funded by NCCAM have included: "Evaluating Yoga for Chronic Low Back Pain," "Yoga as a Treatment for Insomnia," "Yoga: Effect on Attention in Aging and Multiple Sclerosis," and "Yoga for

Treating Shortness of Breath in Chronic Obstructive Pulmonary Disease (COPD)."[1]

A growing number of doctors are following the lead of cardiologist and founder of the Preventive Medicine Research Institute, Dr. Dean Ornish, and incorporating Yoga into their patient recovery programs. According to Dr. Dean Ornish, in his book, Reversing Heart Disease, "Almost all of these (stress reduction) techniques ultimately derive from Yoga." His program is scientifically validated to begin reversing age-related disorders and even severe coronary heart disease without using medications or surgery.

The Beth Israel Medical Center in New York is one of the few facilities in the country to offer personal Yoga therapy instructions for all of its cancer patients. In a research study at the University of California, Los Angeles (UCLA), School of Medicine, a group of people who were sixty or older started doing Yoga postures twice weekly. All the participants had rounded upper backs, which can limit normal movement. Their Yoga regimen was sufficient to reduce their curvatures by 6 percent, increase their walking speeds by 8 percent, and improve their reaches by 18 percent. And many reported that Yoga helped their balance.

Yoga practice has been shown to aid those suffering with chronic pain. A study by the Harbor-UCLA Medical Center (2001) found that patients experiencing chronic pain who also suffer from anxiety, depression, and overuse of medications as a result of their pain improved their symptoms after only four weeks of practicing Yoga. No patients experienced deterioration, and every patient significantly reduced the amount of needed pain medication.[2] Another six-month trial on senior multiple sclerosis patients showed many advantages of Yoga practice for their health.[3]

Yoga is a lifestyle we can follow at every stage of our lives, but especially in our senior years. As our lives have become fast paced over the last one hundred years, because of the technological innovations and specializations, stress levels are rising. The body and mind get overburdened and a sense of unease sets in. Yoga provides a release mechanism for a balance of physical and mental well-being. Yoga is non-competitive. It is not about winning or losing. You go at your own pace with complete freedom. People with limited range of motion or poor flexibility, due to arthritis or otherwise, may benefit the most from Yoga practice, as it can increase flexibility, balance, and strength. Even if you are unable to bend, kneel, or have difficulty getting up and down, modifications are available. You can even practice some Yoga positions entirely in a seated position, in a chair! We all need stress relief, since stress seems to be in everything we do. Yoga and meditation give us the strength to handle life without the sense of pressure and tenseness. It removes imbalance and provides balance.

My friend Alan began to experience back pain after his retirement, and could not play golf, his favorite sport. He was frustrated; he said, "Now I have plenty of time, but I can't play. I was looking forward to my golf practice so much." His wife suggested Yoga exercises to him. He was reluctant at first, but he started some specific Yoga postures for his back (described in Chapter 10). After about three months of Yoga practice, he is back to playing golf and enjoys it more now. He loves the flexibility of all parts of his body. Yoga offers help with other specific health problems, disorders, and conditions too, as we will see in Chapter 10.

I have talked to many people who tell me that they now have better sleep, freedom from fear, freedom from addictions, and relief from anxiety. Beth, a breast cancer survivor, became so weak after her chemotherapy, surgery, and radiation treatment that she could hardly do anything. Then she went into depression and fear of the cancer coming back. Some of us—her friends—suggested

Yoga to her. It was very difficult for her to start the practice, but she said, "What do I have to lose?" She persisted, and now she is fit, active, been healthy for the last ten years, travels a lot, and is active in her church. She has a luster in her skin and a sparkle in her eyes. She has become an advocate of Yoga.

Yoga provides optimum blood supply to various parts of the body by gently stretching muscles and joints as well as massaging various organs. This helps in the flushing out of toxins from every nook and cranny as well as providing nourishment up to the last point. This leads to benefits such as delayed aging, energy, and a remarkable zest for life. Yoga can tone the muscles—muscles that have become flaccid, weak, or flabby are stimulated repeatedly to shed excess flab and flaccidity. Yoga boosts levels of serotonin, endorphins, and dopamine, the three feel-good substances already in your body that make you cheerful, content, and happy. With peace of mind, come better relationships and creativity.

My friend Cathy took pride in running five miles a day, five days a week, when she was in her late forties. She started feeling exhausted and could not sleep at night; after consulting a Yoga teacher, she realized that she was exercising too much for her health. She started a Yoga postures program five days a week. After a couple of months, she recovered her stamina and strength. Now she runs two miles a day, along with her Yoga practice.

It is important to choose the right type of exercise, which is beneficial for the body as well as mind. You should feel energetic and peaceful after you are done with the practice. Yoga is different from other types of exercises in the aspects of connecting our mind and body. We connect the movements of the body and the fluctuations of our mind to the rhythm of our breathing in Yoga. When that happens, our attention moves inward. We become aware of our thoughts without judging them. As we see our habitual thought patterns, we gain more understanding, and then it becomes easier to recognize and modify the patterns.

Sometimes, we all have moments of inner peace, of feeling love, of deep-felt confidence; but for the most part, these are only fleeting experiences that quickly turn into less pleasant ones. Is it possible to train the mind to cultivate these wholesome moments? No doubt, it would change our lives for the better. It will be wonderful to lead our life with peacefulness and inner fulfillment. Yoga offers many different ways to train our body and mind. Yoga includes not only postures (Asanas), but other techniques such as breathing, meditation, and devotion. Practicing any one technique or a combination of all helps. These are very simple and easy to do exercises. By understanding our personality, health conditions, abilities, and limitations, we can choose the type of Yoga that suits us.

The types of Yoga are:

- Yoga of Postures (Asanas or Hatha Yoga) – practice of bodily exercises with postures
- Yoga of Breathing (Pranayama) – breathing methods to strengthen body and mind
- Yoga of Meditation (Dhyana Yoga) - practice for the mind
- Yoga of Devotion (Bhakti Yoga) – practice of prayers, devotion, and worship

We will look at each of these Yoga types in the following chapters.

Our body, mind, and emotions affect each other. If we strengthen one of these, the remaining two can be strong. The key is to understand the relationship of our body, mind, and emotions with the spirit. We can have access to our spirit through our body, mind, and emotions. Yoga provides this access.

The next chapters will provide you with all the information and guidance you need to start a safe and convenient practice in the privacy of your home, where you have flexibility of time. Just set aside thirty minutes of your time and you will be surprised to see how this small amount of time gives you a boost in your energy level for the rest of the day. You will start with centering yourself, then do the warm ups, and then the basic eight postures, which are described in detail in Chapters 4 and 5. After your practice of two weeks, you will add some specific postures to your routine. The practice of the Yoga of breathing, meditation, and devotion can be done any time of the day. The advantage of practicing at home is that you can go at your own pace and take all the time you need without hurry. You can spend a little more time on a specific posture that feels comfortable and eases the stiffness and pain. You can find a variation of a pose. You have more freedom to switch to another pose or to stop. You can do as many repetitions as you like. Having freedom with yourself, spending time with yourself, and connecting to yourself are the activities that really rejuvenate you. It is a practice of nurturing your own self. You will feel relaxed, calm, and energized after your practice. It is always available to you and it is free! You will see more benefits as you continue. The benefits are the greatest reward!

We all want to change for the better. We long for better health, a better outlook, and a better life! The change from our current state to a better state is called transformation. It can happen at our physical level, mental level, or emotional level. When it happens, we gain something of great value, and we feel better because of it.

Valmiki, the author of the great Sanskrit epic "Ramayana" was a highway robber who was transformed into a great poet and author. In his youth, he robbed people and killed them to support his family. One day, a great sage named Narada came into his path. Narada said to him, "You cannot rob me because I don't have anything. And you cannot kill me; I'm one of the immortals." Hearing this, Valmiki became angry. Narada further added, "What you do is wrong and you incur sin. Go ask your family members if they are willing to share the burden of your sins, since they reap some of the benefits of them." He went home and asked them; they all refused to share the burden of his sins. He came back to Narada, asked for forgiveness, and asked him to change him. Narada told him to practice the devotional Yoga of chanting the name of the Lord Rama. Valmiki was determined to change himself and he practiced for a long time. After many years, he heard the voice of God giving him forgiveness and granting him powers. He wrote about Rama, the king of highest virtue and wisdom. The epic "Ramayana" is a wonderful poem with twenty-four thousand verses. It depicts the life of a virtuous person, Rama, and his life of righteousness. The schoolchildren in India learn about Valmiki and "Ramayana" and the transformation. The message they receive is that if a robber can be transformed into a sage, you and I can be improved in our personality and can be transformed into a better person!

We all know that our mind often seems to run wild and that with every emotion it goes into a tailspin. Some emotions like fear or sadness can get trapped in the mind. They do not go away easily. Many times we have experienced anger suddenly, grabbing hold of our mind and staying there. No matter how we try to push it out, it does not move; sometimes it even colors other emotions as well. How do we tame the mind? If we try to control it, it becomes wilder. The yogic way is to free the mind. When the mind is free, it gives up its restlessness and becomes calm. It settles down at a deeper level. At that level, there is only harmony and peace.

You might have had some Yoga classes in the past and you might already know some of the postures. For some reason, you might have stopped your Yoga practice. In that case, after reading this book, you will be able to quickly pick it up and select the postures and other Yoga practices that are beneficial to you at the current state of your body and mind. It will definitely strengthen you now. Getting back to your Yoga practice after a gap is always a joy. I have experienced it a few times. It is like getting back to a mighty storehouse of strength and peace! All you need is an intention to do it.

If you have never tried Yoga, you will start with a clean slate. With your open mind, you will definitely go far, reaping the benefits of your practice.

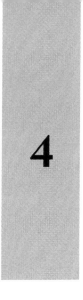

4 Preparing for Yoga practice

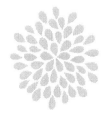

You have made a commitment to practice Yoga! Good decision! Being mentally prepared for Yoga can increase your satisfaction. Having an open mind toward this soothing and nurturing practice will give you a tremendous boost. If you are thinking about starting a Yoga practice but are not sure how to begin, this book will guide you step by step, with all aspects of a safe practice at home. There is no place like your own home and your own space set aside for the practice. For many people, it is not easy to find time and energy to go to a Yoga class at specified times. At home, you have freedom to choose your own time. And with freedom, comes more satisfaction.

The most important thing to keep in mind is to be gentle and kind to yourself when you practice Yoga. The key is to go slowly, especially in the beginning, and to listen to your body. Your body knows what it can do. When it says, "Stop," just stop; do not push it. Yoga is <u>not</u> a competitive sport. If you push too hard, you probably won't enjoy it, and you may hurt yourself. The idea is to explore your limits, not to strive for perfection.

Just remember one thing: "No pain, no gain" is NOT the Yoga way. Due to the low impact of Yoga and the gentle aspect of the motions, there is a very low risk of injury during Yoga practice in comparison to other forms of exercise. In addition, the traditional Yoga poses can be modified according to your health condition. You can even practice while remaining seated in a chair. Doing your Yoga practice in a relaxed way, you will gain strength and flexibility, and you will feel better.

Always consult with your physician before starting your Yoga practice. Experts consider Yoga to be safe but be aware of your physical condition and any limitations in order to prevent injuries. Never practice any Yoga techniques under the influence of alcohol or mind-altering drugs. There are no hard and fast dietary rules necessary to begin the practice of Yoga. One does not have to give up smoking or become a vegetarian. If you are on medications, continue with them, do not stop taking them. Remove your glasses, watches, or any cumbersome jewelry. You can leave your contact lenses on while practicing Yoga. There might be some moaning, groaning, and soreness in the beginning, but the benefits of Yoga outweigh the initial difficulties.

All you will need is a Yoga mat or a flat sheet on carpeted floor to start the practice. Keep a folded towel with you if you need support under your lower back or under your knees, or for your legs. Initially, you might feel that you need support for your arms, legs, and back when doing the poses. You can use bolsters, blocks, props, blankets, or a chair. After a few days of practice, you will discover that you can bend easily and stretch a little more. You will feel warm and fluid inside your body. You will feel more comfortable during the practice. After the practice, you will feel invigorated. Then your daily chores will be done with ease. If you go for a walk, your walk will be more energetic and enjoyable. In other words, what you do every day will have added energy and zest. *These techniques are for prevention and maintenance of good health, gaining strength, and for educational purposes only and should not be used to treat or diagnose a disease.*

The general guidelines for safe Yoga practice include that you need to allow at least two hours after a meal to begin Yoga practice. The stomach should be relatively empty. Yoga practice will flush the toxins from the body so drink plenty of water during the day and keep hydrated. Do not drink water during the practice as you might feel some discomfort in some poses, especially on-your-stomach poses. You will need clothing that is loose fitting and light. It should not be too loose, like a large T-shirt, as some of the poses require that your arms, legs, and neck be free. You do not need to wear socks and shoes but if your feet get cold, you can wear socks.

You will be spending some nurturing time with yourself, so set aside some time free from any distractions. Close the door of your practice room and turn the phones off. Set your attention to the postures and to your body with quiet alertness. Continue with deep breathing throughout the practice. The deep breathing itself will keep your attention on your body and will calm you down. Do not play soft music or radio in the background. Just let your mind follow the awareness of your body. If you are not comfortable with silence during the practice, you can have soft music in the background.

The proper sequence for your entire practice session is to start with centering, warm-ups, and postures, then move on to breathing exercises, and then meditation. Take a few minutes to go into a posture, as described in the next chapter, making sure it is correct. Then hold it, starting with ten seconds. After ten seconds, release it and relax for a few seconds, and then practice it two more times. After two weeks of practice, increase the holding time from ten seconds to twenty seconds, then thirty seconds, working up to sixty seconds. Breathing should be normal and deep during the posture. Some of the postures are done on the right side of the body first and then on the left side; use BOTH sides of the body to gain balance. Holding a posture for ten seconds can be challenging in the beginning for certain conditions, so adjust the time according to your comfort level. Always remember to relax for a few seconds between two poses. Initially you will need twenty minutes for your practice for the beginner's eight postures as described in the next chapter. After two weeks, you might want to add some more postures. Check your body to see how it feels as you add new postures. In Chapter 10, "Yoga for specific conditions," you will see which postures are good for certain health conditions. After reading Chapter 10, you will be able to decide which postures to add to your practice. Have patience with yourself and go forward slowly. As you continue your practice and see the results, your practice time will increase. Yoga practice for half an hour will give you a boost for the entire day.

Another important thing to remember is that there is no rushing. Take your time to learn each pose. As you practice each pose, you are transforming your body, and with this, your mind will be transformed. You will be amazed to see how your body moves, feels, and looks. As you practice each pose, feel the body in that pose and relax all the muscles. Many times we get caught up in checking how our arms and legs are supposed to be, how much distance should be between them, if they are straight or not. Initially, we need to get this figured out, but after that, start feeling the pose. Feel how the stretch inside the body feels, how the muscles feel. Although you are holding the pose, it is not static. Every pose is dynamic because a lot is going on inside the body. The blood is moving easily and smoothly, the blockages are being removed, more oxygen is being received by the cells, toning is going on, toxins are carried away, and in turn, flexibility and strength is created. This will give you tremendous insight into your body and you will be able to visualize the internal you. Your awareness of your body will increase. You will know exactly which part of your body has stiffness or pain. Then you will see the cause and effect of that pain. During certain situations such as colds, flu, or a painful condition or illness, adjust your postures so there is no strain on any part of the body. If you have a fever or a serious illness, do not practice any postures. Practice only breathing exercises and meditation, which will quicken your recovery.

Practicing Yoga will enable you to experience balance and alignment in the body. This is a strong foundation for good health. Yoga postures re-orient the muscles in our body by systematically placing them into challenging stretches. Each pose requires us to hold our body in a unique way. It optimizes flexibility and conscious control. The postures make us aware of many different parts of our body. We usually are not aware of our joints and muscles unless there is pain. In Yoga practice, when we have a good stretch, we become aware of the joints and muscles. When we release a pose, we feel that toning is taking place. Alignment and adjustment take place while we are doing the postures. That is the beauty of Yoga!

There will be a new discovery of "the wisdom of the body" that will give you new insights. A regular practice is needed to see the results. Daily practice is recommended, but if you can find two or three days each week to practice, you will get the benefits of Yoga. The best way is to practice the postures for thirty minutes, then breathing exercises (Pranayama) for fifteen minutes, and then meditation for twenty minutes. You will spend a little over an hour in this practice, and you will see the amazing results it can give you in every area of your life.

5 Yoga of Postures (Asanas - Hatha Yoga)

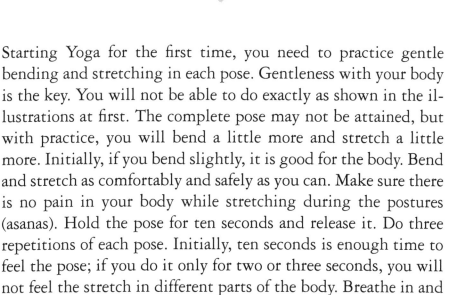

Starting Yoga for the first time, you need to practice gentle bending and stretching in each pose. Gentleness with your body is the key. You will not be able to do exactly as shown in the illustrations at first. The complete pose may not be attained, but with practice, you will bend a little more and stretch a little more. Initially, if you bend slightly, it is good for the body. Bend and stretch as comfortably and safely as you can. Make sure there is no pain in your body while stretching during the postures (asanas). Hold the pose for ten seconds and release it. Do three repetitions of each pose. Initially, ten seconds is enough time to feel the pose; if you do it only for two or three seconds, you will not feel the stretch in different parts of the body. Breathe in and exhale normally during the pose. These eight postures are safe, gentle, and beneficial for overall flexibility for men and women of any age. After a week, you will be happy to see your own progress.

Beginner's sequence of eight basic postures: time – fifteen to twenty minutes

As a beginner, you will start with centering and warm-ups, and then the basic Yoga poses, which are usually a mix of standing and sitting postures, as well as different poses that utilize gentle stretches and bends. A good overall sequence for a practice will be to start with standing poses, then do sitting poses, and then move on to on hands and knees poses, on the stomach poses, on the back poses, twists, inverted poses and lastly the restorative pose of Shavasana. The Sanskrit names of each pose are given in parentheses; you do not need to remember them.

These are the eight beginner's poses; we will see the description of each posture shortly.

1. Standing: Mountain posture (Tadasana) – Standing tall and firm
2. Standing: Hand to foot forward bend posture (Padahastasana)
3. Sitting: Easy posture (Sukhasana) – cross-legged posture
4. Sitting: Forward bend posture (Paschimottanasana)
5. On hands and knees: Cat posture (Marjariasana)
6. Child posture: (Balasana)
7. On the stomach: Cobra posture (Bhujangasana)
8. On the back: Corpse posture – Relaxation pose (Shavasana). This is always the last pose at the end of the posture practice.

Centering

The first step is to sit down in a chair and mentally prepare yourself for the practice. Close your eyes, take a deep breath, and exhale; breathe this way three times. Make a silent intention and affirmation to use your energies to harmonize your body and mind and to expand your self-awareness. It helps to calm yourself, and then you will be ready for the postures.

Warm-ups

1. Stand up straight and tall. Stretch your neck on either side and rotate your head three times.
2. Lift your shoulders up and down three times.
3. Stretch your arms on your sides and rotate them three times.
4. Walk in place for sixty seconds.

Description of postures
1. Mountain posture (Tadasana)

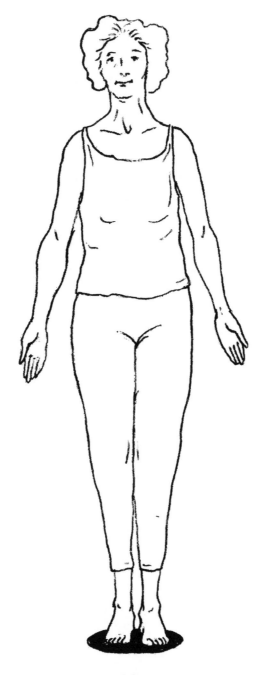

Steps:

1. Stand with both feet close together, keeping the back straight.
2. Keep your arms straight by the sides of your body with palms facing inward and with fingers open.
3. Roll your shoulders back so that your collarbones are widened.
4. Slightly tighten or flex the muscles in your arms, knees, thighs, stomach, and buttocks, maintaining a firm posture.
5. Balance your weight evenly on both feet, standing firm.
6. Stretch your legs, back, and neck upward.
7. Look outward at eye level with your head in a relaxed state.
8. Remain in this pose for 30 seconds, breathing normally.

Benefits:

- The spine gets aligned and the posture is improved.
- The abdomen, thighs, knees, and ankles get strengthened.
- The arms and back are stretched, and receive more circulation.
- This posture improves balance.
- The nervous system gets stronger.

Caution:

If you have a shoulder or back injury, do not roll the shoulders back.

2. Hand to foot forward bend posture (Padahastasana)

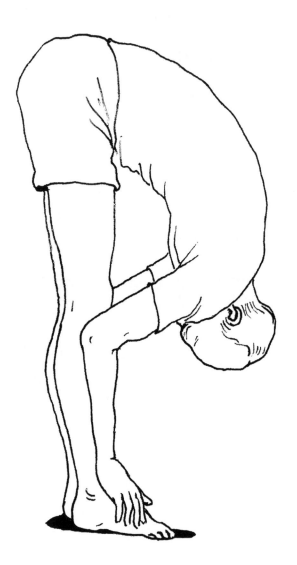

Steps:

1. Stand up straight.
2. Inhale and raise both your arms forward, up to the shoulder level, with palms facing downward.
3. Move your head and neck forward.

40

4. As you exhale, bend down from the waist.
5. Keep your palms straight, bend and try to touch the toes.
6. You may rest your hands gently upon your ankles or thighs, or as far as you are able to stretch downward with a slight bend in your knees.
7. The ideal pose is to place your hands on the toes with your forehead touching the knees. It is the bending that is important; you may not be close to touching the toes initially. Gradually, with practice, you can attain the full pose.
8. Remain in this pose for ten seconds and breathe normally.
9. Slowly inhale and bring your arms up and stand up straight again. Repeat the pose three times.

Benefits:

- In this pose, the abdominal muscles get toned.
- The liver, pancreas, and spleen get activated.
- There is increased blood flow to the brain, pituitary, and thyroid gland, improving metabolism and concentration.
- People suffering from abdominal bloating, acidity, and gastric issues will benefit immensely by practicing this pose.

Caution:

People with a knee injury or a slipped disc in the vertebral column should not practice this pose.

3. Easy posture (Sukhasana) – Cross-legged seated pose

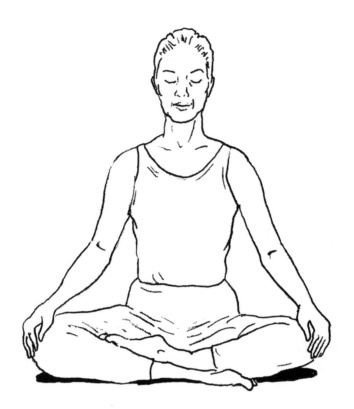

Steps:

1. Begin sitting down on a firm cushion or folded blanket. The hips should be elevated one to two inches from the floor. Cross the legs inward, starting with the left leg in first, and then the right leg. Maintain a comfortable gap between the feet and pelvis.

2. Rest your palms on the knees. Begin to find balance over the pelvis. Prevent the body from leaning back and rounding the spine. Keep the bottom front ribs slightly pulled down. Sit up straight, neither arching forward nor leaning backward.

3. Inhale and lift up through your spine. Exhale and relax the shoulders and collar bone.
4. Relax and close your eyes. Make the tip of your tongue touch the roof of the mouth at the back of your front teeth.
5. Breathe slowly through your nostrils for ten seconds, observing the rhythm of your breath.
6. Repeat crossing the legs the opposite way. Breathe slowly for ten seconds.

Benefits:

- This pose lengthens the spine, establishes spinal alignment, and opens the hips.
- It promotes a grounded feeling and inner calm.
- It amplifies a state of serenity and tranquility, and eliminates anxiety.
- This pose is a great reliever of physical and mental exhaustion, and tiredness.

Caution:

Avoid this pose if you have a recent or chronic knee or hip injury, or inflammation.

4. Sitting with forward bend posture (Paschimottanasana)

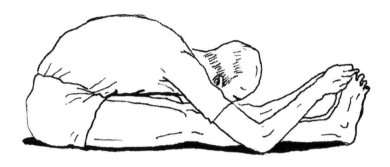

Steps:

1. Sit with your legs straight in front of you, with the back upright.
2. Breathe in and exhale with a slow forward bend at the hips (not at the waist).
3. Bring the chest forward and down slowly, as far as you can.
4. Try to touch or hold your toes with your fingers. Keep your elbows on both sides of the legs. Be sure, not to curve the spine.
5. There should be a slight bend in the knees. Put your head on your knees, if possible. Your head may not go down much, just let it go as much as possible. For support, put a folded towel under your knees.
6. Hold this position for ten seconds and then release it, inhaling, and sitting back.
7. Repeat this pose three times.

Benefits:

- This pose stretches and strengthens the spine, shoulders, and hamstrings.
- It stimulates the liver and kidneys, improving their function.
- It relieves the symptoms of menopause.
- The stretch in the abdominal area improves the appetite and helps digestion.
- Anxiety and fatigue are reduced due to increased circulation.
- It relieves stress and mild depression.

Caution:

If you have a back injury, do not practice this pose.
Avoid this pose if you have diarrhea.

5. On hands and knees: Cat posture (Marjariasana)

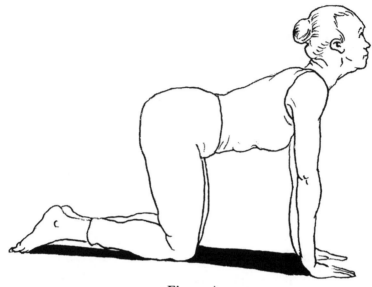

Figure A

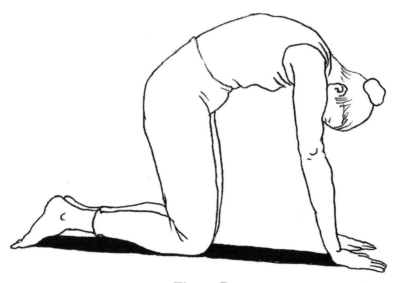

Figure B

Steps:

1. Kneel on your hands and knees, with your hands shoulder width apart and knees hip width apart. Spread your fingers on the floor. Your toes should be touching the floor with heels up. Your wrists should be beneath the shoulders and knees below the hips.
2. Inhale while relaxing the abdomen, keeping your hips straight, with a slight backbend, and with your chin upward looking up with a slight tilt of your head. (Figure A)
3. As you exhale, press down evenly into your hands and contract your abdominal muscles up toward your spine (Figure B). A slight forward spinal curve is needed.
4. Tuck your tailbone under and bring the chin toward the chest. (Figure B)
5. Repeat this arching motion with inhale (Figure A) and exhale. (Figure B)

Benefits:

- This pose increases mobility of the spine and back.
- It strengthens and tones the arms, neck, abdominal muscles, and back muscles.
- It massages the digestive organs and improves digestion.

Caution:

Avoid this pose if you have chronic or recent knee, back, or neck pain.

6. Child posture (Balasana)

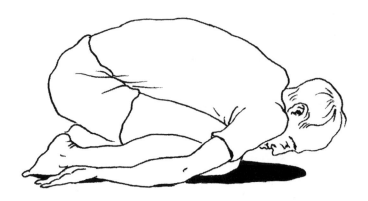

Steps:

1. Sit with your knees apart and legs folded back.
2. Bend forward with hands on either side of your legs and put your head on the floor. You can use a folded towel between the hips and the heels for padding.
3. Hold the pose for ten seconds, breathing normally.
4. Release the pose by slowly sitting upright.
5. Repeat the pose three times.

Benefits:

- This pose stretches the lower back, hips, thighs, knees, and ankles.
- It relaxes the spine and shoulders.
- It relieves neck and back aches.
- The abdominal organs and the chest get massaged in this pose.
- It reduces tension in the body and calms the mind.

Caution:

Avoid this pose if you have knee problems or diarrhea.
This pose is not recommended for individuals with high blood
pressure or ear infections.

7. On the stomach: Cobra posture (Bhujangasana)

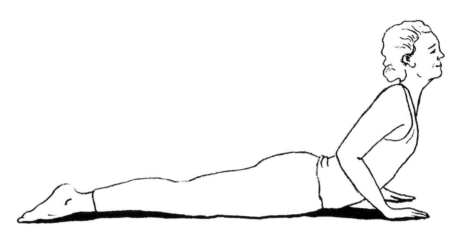

Steps:

1. Lie on your stomach and place your hands on the floor on either side of you.
2. Lift the upper part of your body with your palms down, without lifting your navel from the floor. The elbows should not flay out but remain parallel to the body.

3. Inhale and raise your chest and head, arching your back with a slight backbend. Hold the pose for ten seconds.
4. Exhale while slowly lowering to the floor.
5. Repeat this pose three times.

Benefits:

- This pose stimulates the endocrine system.
- It relieves pain in the back and neck.
- It strengthens the spine and abdominal muscles.
- This pose is effective for women in maintaining the health of the uterus and ovaries.

Caution:

This pose is not recommended for individuals with a hernia or hyperthyroidism.
It should be avoided if you have a peptic ulcer.

8. On the back: Corpse posture – Relaxation pose (Shavasana)

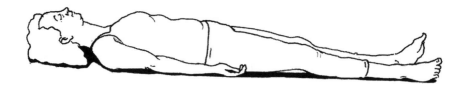

This pose is essential at the end of every Yoga practice.

Steps:

1. Lie down on your back with your legs spread about twelve inches apart.
2. Keep both hands six inches away from your body, palms facing upward.
3. Relax your neck, face, back, and each and every muscle in your whole body. Keep your eyes closed.
4. Inhale and exhale slowly for three minutes.
5. Do not fall asleep, but stay in relaxed awareness.
6. To end the posture, first roll gently with an exhalation onto one side, preferably the right side. Take two or three breaths. With another exhalation press your hands against the floor and lift your body slowly, coming to a sitting position.

Benefits:

- This pose relaxes and rejuvenates the body, mind, and spirit.
- It reduces stress and tension, and calms you down.
- It brings down blood pressure and heart rate.
- It balances and integrates the energies in the body at the end of your Yoga practice.

Caution:

Do not sleep while in this pose. Keep your attention on your breathing.

6 Additional postures

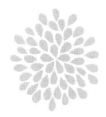

These additional postures include standing postures, sitting postures, twist postures, on-hands-and-knees postures, on-the-stomach postures, on back postures, and inverted postures. Each posture includes the steps, benefits, and cautionary notes. The best way to decide which postures to practice is to read the following chapters in this book, especially Chapter 10, which gives information about specific health conditions and which postures will be good for those conditions. Remember, the last posture to practice is the Relaxation pose (Shavasana).

I. Standing postures:

1. Chair posture (Utkatasana)

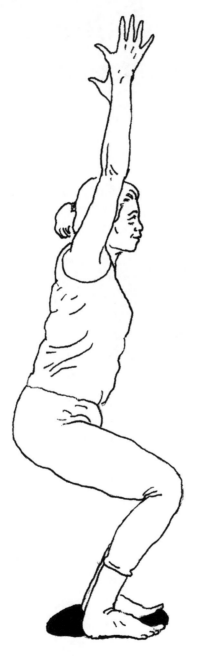

Steps:

1. Stand up straight with your feet together and with your arms raised up.
2. Bend the knees and lower the hips until the thighs are parallel to the floor. The spine should remain straight.
3. Hold this pose for ten seconds and breathe normally.
4. Stand up straight.
5. Repeat this pose for two more times.

Benefits:

- This pose strengthens the spine, hips, hamstrings, thighs, and knees.
- The chest, shoulders, and abdomen get stretched and get more circulation.
- It helps with arthritis of the knees.
- It stimulates the heart and the diaphragm.

Caution:

This pose is not recommended for individuals with low blood pressure and headaches.
If you have knee, hip, or ankle problems, do not practice this pose.

2. Warrior 1 posture (Virabhadrasana 1)

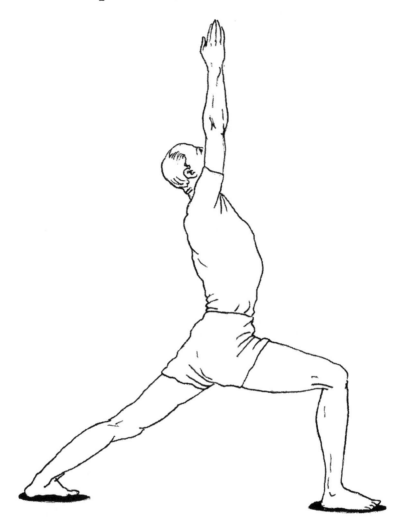

Steps:

1. Stand up straight. Step your left foot back three to four feet and turn it 45 degrees. It should be straight.
2. Bend your right foot at 90 degrees at the knee and keep slightly more pressure on your right foot.
3. You should be facing forward, in the direction of the right foot, with your hips pointing forward.

4. Lift your arms up straight with your palms facing inward.

5. Hold the pose for ten seconds while inhaling and exhaling.

6. Lower your arms, bring your feet together, and stand up straight.

7. Do the same pose on the other side (right foot back, left foot in the front), hold for ten seconds.

8. Repeat this sequence (steps 1 through 7) two more times.

Benefits:

- This pose strengthens the shoulders, arms, and thighs.
- It stretches the groin, lower back, abdomen, and ankles.
- The digestive organs get stretched and stimulated.
- It expands the chest and lungs.
- It improves balance for the whole body.

Caution:

Avoid this pose if you have high blood pressure or a heart condition.
It is not recommended for individuals with shoulder, knee, or back problems.

3. Warrior2 posture (Virabhadrasana 2)

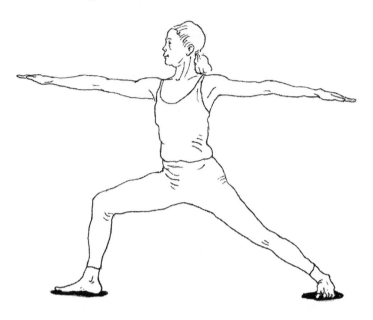

Steps:

1. Stand up straight. Step your left foot back three to four feet and turn it 45 degrees. It should be straight.
2. Bend your right foot at 90 degrees at the knee and keep slightly more pressure on your right foot.
3. You should be facing forward, in the direction of your right foot, with your hips pointing the side.
4. Lift your arms up straight and parallel to the floor. Your left arm is in the same direction as your left foot.
5. Hold the pose for ten seconds while inhaling and exhaling.

6. Lower your arms, bring your feet together, and stand up straight.
7. Do the same pose on the other side (right foot back and left foot in the front), hold for ten seconds.
8. Repeat this sequence (steps 1 through 7) two more times.

Benefits:

- This pose strengthens the legs, thighs, and back.
- It stretches the groin, chest, and shoulders.
- The digestive organs get stretched and stimulated.
- It relieves back pain.

Caution:

Avoid this pose if you have high blood pressure or a heart condition.
It is not recommended for people with shoulder, knee, or back problems.

4. Triangle posture (Trikonasana)

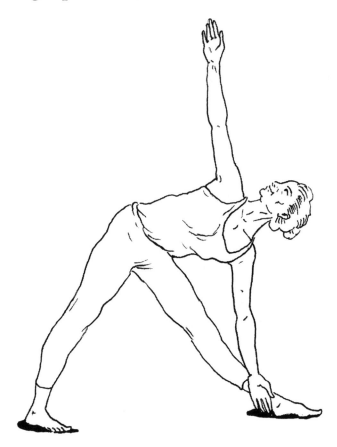

Steps:

1. Stand with your feet three feet apart.
2. Move your left foot outward at an angle of 90 degrees.
3. Move your right foot inward at an angle of 45 degrees. Both legs should be straight, without locking the knees.
4. Raise your arms outstretched until they are parallel to the floor.
5. Move your right arm up and left arm down toward your ankle. If you cannot reach the ankle, reach up to the knee.

6. Turn your head up, looking at your right hand.
7. Hold the pose for ten seconds.
8. Bring the arms back to the outstretched position.
9. Repeat two more times.
10. Do the same pose on the other side; hold for ten seconds each time.

Benefits:

- This pose strengthens the legs, groin, and back.
- It stretches the arms, chest, shoulders, and abdominal area.
- It helps remove fat from the thighs and waist.
- It helps digestion and stimulates appetite.

Caution:

This pose is not recommended for people with back problems.

II. Sitting postures:

1. Auspicious Posture (Bhadrasana)

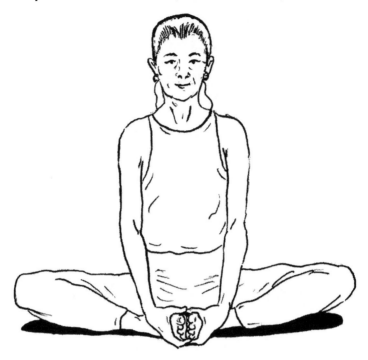

Steps:

1. Sit straight and erect with legs bending at the knees in the front.
2. Join the soles of your feet together and keep your heels and toes together.
3. Clasp your fingers around your toes.
4. Draw your feet inward little by little, and bring the knees closer to the floor.
5. Hold the pose for ten seconds, with inhale and exhale.
6. Release your fingers from the toes.
7. Repeat the pose for two more times.

Benefits:

- This pose restores elasticity to stiff knees, hips, and ankle joints.
- It has a beneficial effect on the kidneys, prostate, and urinary bladder.
- It strengthens the groin and pelvis.
- It massages the lower abdomen and improves digestion.

Caution:

Do not force the knees down; just relax the thighs.
This pose is not recommended to people with hip or spinal injuries.

2. Bending knees and sitting on heels (Vajrasana)

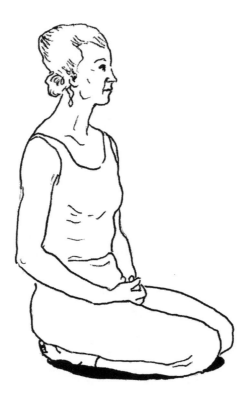

Steps:

1. Slowly kneel down, bend your knees, and release your toes on the floor.
2. Rest your buttocks on the soles of your feet. If needed, use a folded towel under the ankles or in between the hips and ankles.
3. Place your palms downward on the knees.
4. Keep your spine and head straight.
5. Inhale and exhale slowly for thirty seconds.

Benefits:

- This pose improves and aids digestion.
- It conditions the pelvic muscles, thighs, knees, and ankles.
- It strengthens the heart and chest.
- It tones the legs and thighs.

Caution:

This pose is not recommended for people with knee injuries or ankle problems.

3. Lotus posture (Padmasana) - classic Yoga pose

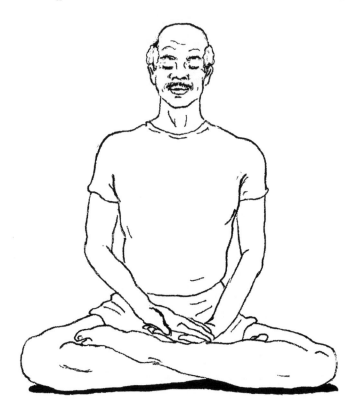

Steps:

1. Sit on the floor with both legs stretched out in front of you.
2. Bend your right knee; hold your right foot with both hands and place it on top of your left thigh. Bring your right heel close to the navel.
3. Bend your left knee; hold your left foot with both hands, and place it on top of your right thigh. Bring the heel close to the naval.
4. Both knees should be touching the floor and the soles of both feet pointed upward.
5. The spine, neck, and head are held straight.

6. Rest your hands on your heels, one hand on top of the other hand or rest them on your knees, palms facing downward or upward.
7. Breathe in and out for thirty seconds.
8. Release the pose, reverse the leg positions, and hold the pose for thirty seconds.

Benefits:

- This pose creates natural balance in body and mind.
- It stretches the groin, knees, thighs, and ankles.
- This restful pose straightens the spine, back, and neck.
- It reduces lower back pain.
- It reduces tension and increases mobility in the body.
- It increases circulation in the lumbar area and the abdominal area.
- It has a relaxing effect on the nervous system and it reduces blood pressure.
- This stable pose, generating steadiness and calmness, is good for meditation.

Caution:

This pose is not recommended if you have knee injury, knee pain, or sciatica.
If your legs feel pain in this pose, sit in the Easy pose (Sukhasana) as described in the last chapter.

III. Twist postures:

1. Spinal twist (Matsyendrasana)

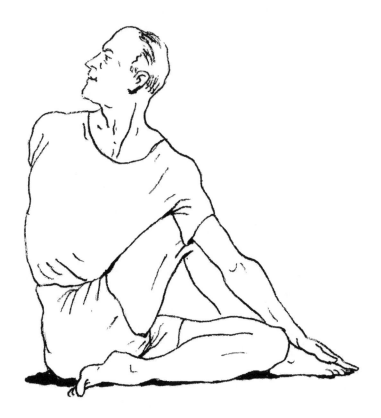

Steps:

1. Sit on the floor with your legs straight out in front of you. Bend the left leg at the knee.
2. Step your right foot over your left leg, just outside the left hip. Place it flat on the floor. Your right knee should point upward.
3. Twist your torso on the right side and set your upper left arm on the outside of your right thigh.

4. Place your right hand against the floor just behind your left buttock. Bring this hand around your waist and make your fingers touch the left thigh.
5. Twist evenly throughout the spine.
6. Breathe normally and hold the pose for thirty seconds.
7. Release the pose slowly.
8. Now do the same pose on the other side of the body and hold for thirty seconds.

Benefits:

- This posture stimulates the liver, pancreas, kidneys, spleen, and colon.
- It adjusts and tones the vertebral column, neck, and shoulders.
- It relieves tension in the back.
- Circulation is improved in the spine and back.
- It helps abdominal organs and improves digestion.
- It trims fat accumulation in the middle part of the body.
- It increases flexibility in the pelvis, hips, and legs.

Caution:

This pose is not recommended for people with neck or back problems.

2. Lying-twist (Jathara-Parivatasana)

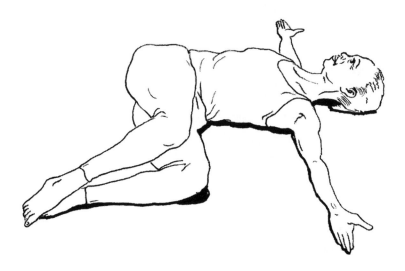

Steps:

1. Lie on your back with your legs straight and your arms extended on each side.
2. Bring both legs up together and bend them slightly at the knees. Bring both legs down touching the floor on the left side and move your face toward the right, giving a twist to the body.
3. Hold the pose for thirty seconds.
4. Straighten the legs slowly and let the back touch the floor.
5. Repeat this pose (steps 1 and 2) on the other side.
6. Hold the pose for thirty seconds.

Benefits:

- This posture stretches the spine, shoulders, arms, and legs.
- It stimulates the bladder, kidneys, and intestines.
- It improves digestion and circulation.

Caution:

Be careful with twisting your body if you have chronic back pain, disc injuries, or osteoporosis.

IV. On hands-and-knees postures:

1. Downward facing dog (Adho Mukhasana)

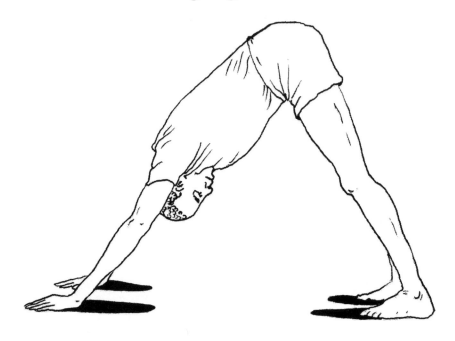

Steps:

1. Come to your hands and knees on the floor. Place your palms in the front about eighteen inches apart.
2. Raise your hips up until your legs and your arms are straight.
3. Place your feet flat on the floor about hip-width apart, with toes facing forward.
4. Move your head down between your arms, looking downward. Let the head hang freely.

5. Keep the back flat.
6. Hold the pose for thirty seconds, breathing in and out.
7. Release the pose by bending the knees and bringing hips down.

Benefits:

- This posture builds strength in arms, wrists, and legs.
- It tones the muscles in the back and the abdomen.
- The chest, ribs, and the calves get a good stretch.
- It stimulates the brain and nervous system and improves memory and concentration.
- It relieves lower back pain.

Caution:

Do not try a complete stretch if you have back or shoulder problems.

V. On the stomach postures:

1. Bow posture (Dhanurasana)

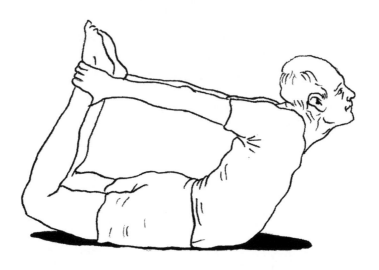

Steps:

1. Lie on your stomach.
2. Reach both hands back and grasp your ankles.
3. Draw your torso and legs up at the same time.
4. Only your abdomen should be touching the floor.
5. Hold the pose for thirty seconds.
6. Release the pose by bringing your hands and torso down.

Benefits:

- This pose expands the chest and lungs and improves respiratory conditions.
- It increases circulation to heart, abdomen, back, and legs.
- It tones the spine, neck, thighs, and arms.

- It helps to regulate prostate gland and ovaries.
- It strengthens liver, kidneys, pancreas, and spleen.
- It improves digestion and oxygen intake.
- It reduces abdominal fat.

Caution:

This pose is not recommended for the people with a peptic ulcer, hernia, or gastrointestinal disorders.

If you have lower back problems, do not practice this pose.

2. Locust pose (Shalabhasana)

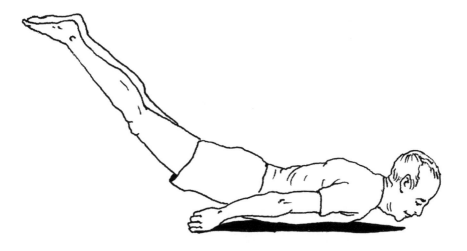

Steps:

1. Lie on your stomach with arms stretched by the sides.
2. Raise your legs up, keeping your knees straight.
3. Rest your chin on the floor.
4. Your navel should be on the floor and not raised.
5. Hold the pose for ten seconds, breathing normally.
6. Release the pose slowly, rest for ten seconds, and practice it two more times.

Benefits:

- This pose strengthens the muscles of the pelvis, thighs, legs, and lower back.
- It massages the intestinal organs and improves digestion
- It tones the neck, arms, and shoulders.
- It can relieve sciatica pain and lower back pain.

Caution:

If you cannot lift your legs up much, try to lift them slightly, about six inches off the floor.

This pose is not recommended for people with lower back or spine injuries.

VI. On the back postures:

1. Leg raise (Urdhva Prasarita Padasana)

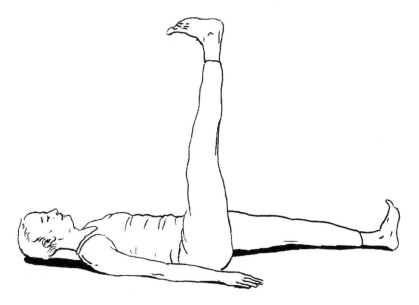

Steps:

1. Lie on your back with your legs straight on the floor.
2. Slowly raise both legs together until they are straight up, at 90 degrees.
3. Keep your arms by your sides, palms facing down.
4. Do not bend your knees and make sure your lower back remains flat on the floor.
5. Hold the pose for thirty seconds, breathing in and out.
6. Release the pose by bringing the legs down slowly.

Benefits:

- This pose strengthens the abdominal organs and muscles and improves digestion.
- It tones the legs, thighs, and ankles.
- Blood circulation increases in the abdominal area, pelvic area, and the back.
- It enables the spine to lengthen.
- It trims the waist and thighs.

Caution:

If you cannot raise both feet, raise one foot and then the other foot.
If you have lower back injury or pain, do not practice this pose.

2. Fish pose (Matsyasana)

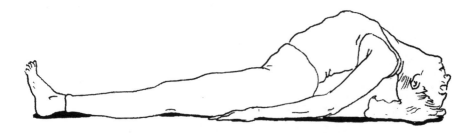

Steps:

1. Lie on your back with your feet straight together.
2. Place your arms on your sides with your palms facing downward and your elbows on the floor.
3. Lift your upper body into a backward bend with head bending backward and slowly touching the floor.
4. Your buttocks should remain on the floor.
5. Your back should be arching up, and not touching the floor.
6. Hold the pose for thirty seconds, breathing in and out slowly.
7. Release the pose by straightening your head first and then your upper body.

Benefits:

- Your spine, back, shoulders, and neck get a good stretch with this pose.
- The abdomen and chest get expanded, stretched, and strengthened.
- The throat and the thyroid gland get stimulated.
- It encourages deep breathing.
- It strengthens the kidneys, intestines, and pelvic organs.

Caution:

This pose is not recommended for people who suffer from a heart condition, a peptic ulcer, back problems, or a hernia.
If you feel any strain in your back, necks, or head, stop practicing it.

3. Side-to-side roll with knees to chest (Pavanmuktasana)

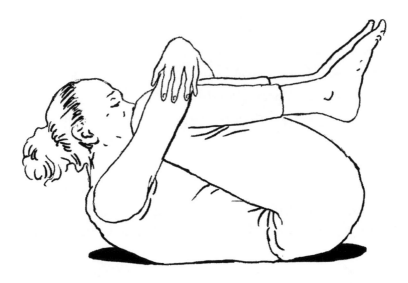

Steps:

1. Lie on your back with your legs straight.
2. Raise your left knee to your chest and then raise your right knee to your chest.
3. Hold both knees together with your arms around them.
4. Lift your neck up about two inches.
5. Roll from side to side slowly while in this pose.
6. Practice for sixty seconds.

Benefits:

- This pose massages the colon, small intestine, liver, and all digestive organs, and relieves gas from the stomach.
- It regulates and normalizes hydrochloric acid levels in the stomach.
- It helps with sciatica and joint pain by creating more circulation.
- It massages the back, hips, thighs, and legs.
- It improves the functioning of the heart and lungs.
- It reduces obesity and excess fat around the stomach.

Caution:

This pose is not recommended if you have back problems, back pain, or slipped disc.

4. Bridge pose (Setu Bandhasana)

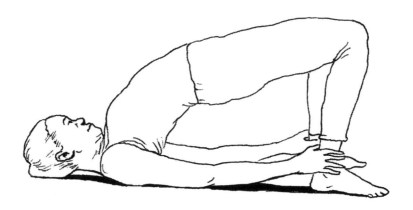

Steps:

1. Lie on your back with arms straight and palms facing down.
2. Bend your knees, lift them up and bring your feet close to the hips.
3. Lift your upper body while keeping the legs straight down. Your spine should peel up off the mat.
4. Your back should not touch the floor, only your shoulders should touch the floor.
5. Keep your head on the floor and hold your ankles with your fingers.
6. Hold the pose for thirty seconds while breathing in and out slowly.
7. Release the pose by bringing your back to the floor slowly and then stretching your legs.

Benefits:

- This pose is beneficial to the individuals with blocked arteries.
- It stretches the chest, spine, neck, knees, and legs.
- The shoulders, arms, and back get strengthened.
- This pose stimulates the liver, pancreas, intestines, colon, lungs, and thyroid.
- It increases blood circulation in the entire body.
- It relieves the symptoms of menopause.
- It is therapeutic for high blood pressure, asthma, and osteoporosis

Caution:

Avoid this pose if you have a neck, shoulder, or back problem. For a tight shoulder or neck, use a towel under your head and neck.

VII. Inverted postures:

1. Shoulder stand (Sarvangasana)

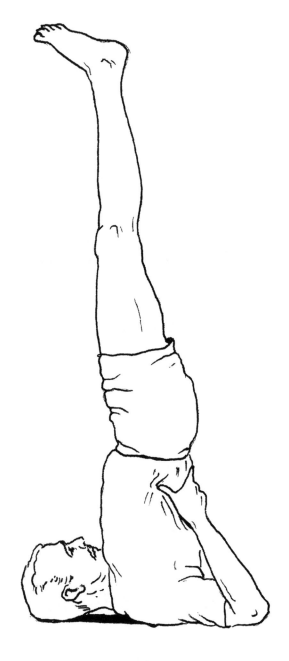

Steps:

1. Lie on your back with your legs straight.
2. Lift your legs slowly up, legs together, first 30 degrees up, then 60 degrees, and then 90 degrees.
3. Straighten your legs, lift your buttocks, and support the back of your trunk with your palms.
4. Keep your elbows on the floor, straight in line with your shoulders.
5. Lift your legs high up so that your heels, hips, and shoulders are aligned in a straight line. Adjust them as much as you can.
6. Your body should be resting on your shoulders and not on your back or neck.
7. Hold the pose for thirty seconds, breathing in and out normally.
8. Release the pose slowly by lowering your back first and then your legs.

Benefits:

- This pose reverses the effects of gravity. It directs the blood circulation from the entire lower body toward the heart.
- It reduces the pressure on the legs and reduces or prevents varicose veins.
- It helps the lungs by carrying more oxygen to all of its parts.
- The brain benefits by more blood flowing toward it.
- The thyroid gland gets stimulated.
- The back, shoulders, and the neck get strengthened.
- It invigorates the nervous and digestive systems.
- It promotes good sleep.

Caution:

This pose is not recommended for people with heart problems, high blood pressure, kidney problems, or neck injuries.
If you have back pain or knee pain, practice this pose cautiously.

2. Plow posture (Halasana)

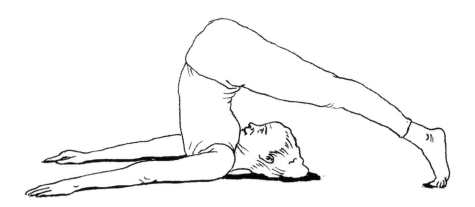

Steps:

1. Lie on your back with your legs straight and arms by your sides.
2. Raise your legs up and bend at the hips, making the legs move toward your head and further.
3. Keep your legs fully stretched and move your legs as far as they can go.
4. Keep your arms flat on the floor.
5. Your chin should touch your chest
6. Hold the pose for thirty seconds, breathing in and out normally.
7. Release the pose by supporting your back with your hands and slowly lowering your torso.

Benefits:

- This pose strengthens the spine, hamstrings, back, and neck.
- It stretches each one of the vertebrae, stretching every spinal muscle and ligament.
- The abdominal organs get stimulated and digestion gets improved.
- It relieves the symptoms of menopause.
- It strengthens the shoulders, arms, legs, and feet.
- The thyroid gland gets stimulated.
- This pose is therapeutic for sinusitis and headaches.

Caution:

This pose should be avoided if you have high blood pressure, asthma, or neck problems.
If you have back pain, practice this pose cautiously.

The Sun Salutations (Surya Namaskar)

The Sun Salutation is an energizing sequence that integrates the body, mind, and breath. It uses our whole being to bow to the Sun, to reach up to the sky, bow forward to the Earth in prostration, and get back up with gratitude. It is a process of offering our salutation to the divine, represented by the Sun, as the source of light and remover of darkness. All life on Earth depends on the Sun's energy. The Sun Salutation gives us an opportunity to capture that energy through our breath. We follow the breath as we go into the next pose in the sequence. The Sun Salutations activate and revitalize every part of the body and illumine the mind. It is an alternate way of the practice of Yoga Asanas because it includes many of the poses that are described previously.

The Sun salutations exercise can be done by itself, without any of the other poses that are described previously. Start with three rounds for the first week and then add one round each week, and go up to twelve rounds. After four or five sequences, our breathing becomes faster, we get more oxygen, the blood circulation increases and the heart rate rises. During this practice, we are continuously bending and stretching, with the forward and backward movements of our spine, arms, legs, abdomen, back, and neck. Every part of the body gets exercised. After a few more rounds, we get a good workout. In this sequence, you may not be able to reach the desired bend and stretch completely. Do all bending and stretching as much as you can comfortably, without pain.

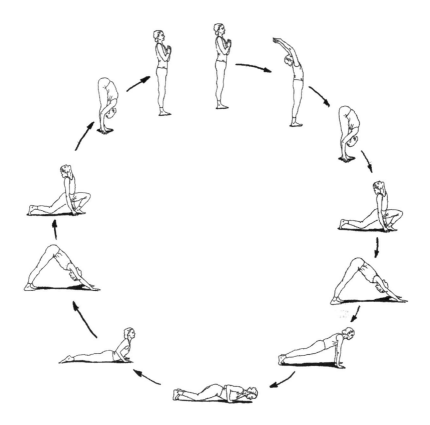

Steps:

1. Begin by standing up straight with your hands in prayer position (both palms joining together, in front of your chest).
2. Inhale and raise your arms up.
3. As you exhale, bend forward slowly and touch your toes with your fingers, touching your head to your knees.
4. Inhale and step your left leg back, with the right knee bent and with your hands on the floor on both sides.
5. As you exhale, step the right leg back and go in Downward Dog pose.
6. Inhale and go into plank position (your whole body is up, straight, and on the same level from the floor, with only hands and toes touching the floor).

7. Exhale and lower yourself flat on the floor with your stomach, knees, and forehead touching the floor.
8. Inhale and lift your chest up in Cobra pose, supporting the body with both arms.
9. Exhale and do the Downward Dog pose.
10. Inhale and step your left foot forward and then your right foot forward.
11. Exhale and bring your head to your knees with your hands to the toes.
12. Inhale, stand with your arms raised, then exhale and lower your arms into prayer position.

Benefits:

- The Sun Salutations provide a profound stretch for the entire body.
- The alternate forward and backward bending creates flexibility in all parts of the body.
- It activates the digestive system by alternate stretching and compression of the digestive organs.
- It tones up the nervous system and improves memory.
- It normalizes the activity of the endocrine glands, especially the thyroid gland.
- It reduces obesity and fat accumulation in the middle part of the body.
- It makes the spine, back, thighs, and legs strong.
- It reduces chemical dependency and addictions.

Caution:

This sequence of twelve postures is not recommended if you have high blood pressure or heart conditions.
If you have a back problem, practice the Sun Salutations carefully.

❖ ❖ ❖

7 Yoga of Breathing (Pranayama)

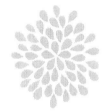

Pranayama is a Sanskrit word that means "control of prana." Prana is life force, or the vital energy that we maintain through our breathing. Breathing absorbs prana into the body. This life force pervades the entire body. Breathing is the only means of supplying the body with oxygen, which is vital to our survival. It is the connecting link between the body and mind. Yoga teaches us the proper way to breathe. It teaches us that using this breath control we can still the mind and reach a higher state of awareness. The practice of Pranayama rewards us with a steady mind, self-control, strong will power, sound judgment, and good health in our daily life.

We can survive without food for weeks and without water for days, but without oxygen, our brain will suffer cellular damage within minutes and we will die. Our brain requires more oxygen than our other organs. The hundred billion cells in our brain continuously use oxygen to stoke the mental fire. However, the brain is such a heavy user of oxygen, it is particularly susceptible to oxidative damage. If our brain does not get enough oxygen, the result is mental sluggishness, depression, anxiety, negative thoughts and behaviors, and decline in the functioning in our body. The Yoga of Breathing gives us more oxygen and energy, and in turn, more vitality. Prana and mind have an intricate link. If there is a fluctuation in one, there will be a fluctuation in the other. If one is balanced, the other will be in a state of balance. The practice of Pranayama is the preparation for the Yoga of Meditation.

Several research studies have reported that the Pranayama techniques are useful in stress related disorders, in relieving the symptoms of asthma, and in reducing pain and discomfort. The breathing process has a direct connection to our brain, our nervous system, and our emotional responses. Erratic breathing creates erratic impulses in the brain and disturbed states in the body. By becoming aware of our breathing, we can balance our whole system. Proper breathing can strengthen our sympathetic and parasympathetic nervous systems. During the Pranayama practice, our mind is steady and aware and it is not moving from thought to thought. Breathing is the only major life process in our body that is controlled through both the central nervous system and autonomic nervous system. It goes on when we are asleep through our autonomic nervous system. With the practice of Pranayama, we can control it for our benefit. Pranayama emphasizes deepening and lengthening our breath. This stimulates the relaxation response—the opposite of the fight-or-flight adrenaline rush of the stress response. It helps us to stay connected to the present moment. In a study on senior volunteers, after thirty days of practicing Pranayama, some reduction in triglycerides, free fatty acids, and LDL cholesterol, along with significant elevation of HDL cholesterol was observed in men and free fatty acids were reduced in women.

Breathing is one of the most remarkable functions of the anatomy and physiology of the body. It is the only biological activity that can be brought under full conscious control and it also functions autonomically twenty-four hours a day.

How is your breathing?

Our breathing is generally shallow and fast. It is that way because we are in a hurry most of the time. It becomes our habit to focus our attention on other things than our own breathing. Shallow breathing does not exercise the lungs enough and they lose their function, causing further reduction in vitality. We do not take in enough oxygen and we do not eliminate enough carbon dioxide, resulting in low energy levels and tiredness. The basic factors that affect our breathing are our lifestyle, diet, desires, thoughts, and emotions. As we balance our breathing, these factors become harmonized and balanced in our life. The breath plays a major role in many cases of excess anxiety. When we have a feeling of anxiety, the breath becomes shallow, rapid, and constricted, which in turn reinforces our nervous system's state of anxiety.

The first step is to become aware of our breathing. Then we can regulate it better. In order to check your breathing, sit comfortably in a chair and close your eyes. Breathe in and out. Notice your inhalation and exhalation.

- Are you taking in air enough to expand your lungs fully?
- Do you feel your rib cage move upward?
- Does your stomach move when you inhale?
- As you exhale, does most of the air go out of the lungs?
- Is your breathing quick and fast, or slow and deep?

The lungs should expand to their full capacity when you breathe in and the inhalation should be long and deep. Your stomach should expand outward. The ribs should expand outward. The lungs should be filled fully without any strain or discomfort. As you exhale, the stomach should relax completely and the lungs should expel as much air as possible. Practice this deep breathing for a few minutes with a complete focus on it. This kind of breathing is used in the practice of different types of Pranayama that are described in this chapter.

Getting ready to practice Pranayama:

The best way to practice is to sit on the floor, on a mat or a folded towel. Sit in Easy pose (Sukhasana as described in Chapter 5) or in Lotus pose (Padmasana as described in Chapter 6) with your back, head, and neck straight. If you have knee or back pain and you cannot sit on the floor, you can practice sitting in a chair with your back and head straight. Blow your nose before starting the practice. Keep the mouth closed and breathe through your nose during the practice. Close your eyes so your mind can focus on your breathing. The practice of Pranayama needs to be done once or twice daily. If you are under tension or stress, or feeling uncomfortable or anxious in any situation, or are agitated or angry, practicing Pranayama (any breathing exercise described in this chapter) for two or three minutes will calm you down and you will gain self-control. Pranayama is best practiced right after the Postures (Asanas), without breaking the flow of awareness. Pranayama is a prerequisite for successful meditation.

Types of Pranayama

Pranayama is a practice of controlled inhalation and exhalation, combined with retention of breath. Retention is an important part because it allows time to assimilate the energy from breath. There is an exchange of oxygen and carbon dioxide in the cells.

There are seven commonly used forms of Pranayama:

- Alternate Nostril breathing (Nadi shodhana)
- Right Nostril breathing (Sun breath or Surya-bheda)
- Left Nostril breathing (Moon breath)
- Victorious breathing (Ujjayi)
- Bellows breathing (Bhastrika)
- Cooling breathing (Sheetali)
- Humming bee breathing (Bhramari)

1. Alternate Nostril breathing (Nadi shodhana)

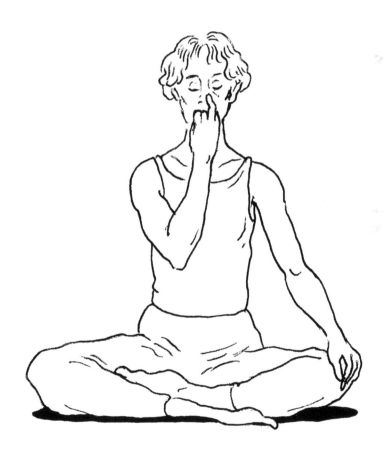

Nadi is a Sanskrit word for a channel in the body and shod-hana means purification. Pranayama provides purification of all channels in the body through the breath.

Steps:

1. Sit comfortably upright, with your back, neck, and head in a straight line and close your eyes.
2. With your right-hand thumb, close your right nostril.
3. Slowly inhale through your left nostril for a slow count of four (1, 2, 3, 4).
4. With your right hand ring finger, close your left nostril.
5. Exhale slowly through your right nostril for a slow count of four (1, 2, 3, 4).
6. Inhale through your right nostril for a slow count of four (1, 2, 3, 4).
7. With the right-hand thumb, close the right nostril.
8. Exhale through the left nostril for a slow count of four (1, 2, 3, 4).
9. This is one round. Practice ten rounds (steps 2 through 8).
10. Optional step – After practicing this kind of breathing for a week, try to hold your breath for four seconds after each inhalation and after each exhalation.

Tips:

1. If your right hand and arm get tired, support the elbow with the palm of your left hand.
2. Make sure your head is not tilting in any direction and remains steady.
3. Practice ten rounds in the beginning for a week and then increase the rounds slowly by adding one round per week. Go up to fifteen rounds for your regular practice.

Benefits:

- Alternate Nostril breathing balances both the right and left hemispheres of the brain. They are associated with "thinking" and "feeling" parts. It also balances the electrical activity in the brain.
- It reduces anxiety and brings calmness.
- Focusing on breathing makes the mind steady, calm, and alert.
- It increases the flow of oxygen in the body and purifies the blood.
- It clears the nasal passages and sinuses.
- It gives relief from allergies, headaches, and depression.
- It lowers the blood pressure.
- The nervous system gets soothed and functions more efficiently.
- The quality of sleep gets better. The sleep becomes deep and restful.
- It cleanses the lungs, and the lung capacity increases.
- The effects of asthma can be reduced tremendously.
- The feeling of tiredness is replaced by more energy.

Caution:

If you have a cold or your nasal passages are blocked for any reason, do not practice the Alternate Nostril breathing.

Do not force your breath; it needs to flow slowly.

2. Right Nostril breathing (Sun breathing – Surya Bheda)

The common technique used in Yoga is breathing through one nostril at a time. Medical research in electroencephalogram (EEG) studies of the electrical impulses of the brain have shown that breathing through one nostril results in increased activity on the opposite side of the brain. Experts suggest that the regular practice of breathing through one nostril may help improve communication between the right and left side of the brain. Studies have also shown that this increased brain activity is associated with better performance and enhancement in cognitive performance.

Surya Bheda consists of using the right nostril for inhalation. The right side channels in the body represent the Sun or vital energy. This breathing stimulates the sympathetic nervous system and the left hemisphere of the brain. It makes the body ready for action. Practice method 1 or method 2 or both.

Method 1:

Steps:

1. Sit comfortably upright with your back, neck, and head erect and close your eyes.
2. With your right hand ring finger, close your left nostril.
3. Slowly inhale through your right nostril for a slow count of four (1, 2, 3, 4).
4. With your right hand thumb, close your right nostril.
5. Exhale slowly through your left nostril for a slow count of four (1, 2, 3, 4).
6. This is one round. Practice ten rounds (steps 2 through 5).
7. Optional step – After practicing this kind of breathing for a week, try to hold your breath for four seconds after each inhalation and after each exhalation.

Method 2:

Steps:

1. Sit comfortably upright with your back, neck, and head erect and close your eyes.

2. With your right hand ring finger, close your left nostril.
3. Slowly inhale through your right nostril for a slow count of four (1, 2, 3, 4).
4. Slowly exhale through your right nostril for a slow count of four (1, 2, 3, 4).
5. This is one round. Practice ten rounds (steps 3 and 4).
6. After practicing this kind of breathing for a week, try to hold your breath for four seconds after each inhalation and after each exhalation.

Benefits:

- Right Nostril breathing generates energy in the body and creates heat in the body.
- It increases digestive fire, improves appetite, and balances the digestive system.
- This breathing exercise gradually increases concentration.
- It makes the immune system stronger.
- It gives relief from asthma and colds.

Caution:

This breathing exercise is not recommended for people who suffer from excessive acidity, epilepsy, or heart ailments.

3. Left Nostril breathing (Moon breathing)

The left nostril is connected to the right hemisphere in the brain, which can activate the parasympathetic nervous system. The parasympathetic nervous system counteracts the effects of stress. It calms you down, slows the heart rate, lowers blood pressure, relaxes you, and runs the automatic tasks of digestion, elimination, healing, and sleep cycle.

Method 1:

Steps:

1. Sit comfortably upright with your back, neck, and head erect and close your eyes.
2. With your right hand thumb, close your right nostril.
3. Slowly inhale through your left nostril for a slow count of four (1, 2, 3, 4).
4. With your right hand ring finger, close your left nostril.
5. Exhale slowly through your right nostril for a slow count of four (1, 2, 3, 4).
6. This is one round. Practice ten rounds (steps 2 through 5).
7. Optional step – After some practice of this kind of breathing for a week, try to hold your breath for four seconds after each inhalation and after each exhalation.

Method 2:

Steps:

1. Sit comfortably upright with your back, neck, and head erect, and close your eyes.
2. With your right hand thumb, close your right nostril.
3. Slowly inhale through your left nostril for a slow count of four (1, 2, 3, 4).
4. Exhale slowly through your left nostril for a slow count of four (1, 2, 3, 4).
5. This is one round. Practice ten rounds (steps 3 and 4).
6. Optional step – After practicing for a week, hold your breath for four seconds after each inhalation and exhalation.

Benefits:

- Left Nostril breathing helps with insomnia. It is an effective way to wind down, relax, and go to sleep.
- It clears acne and skin disorders.

Caution:

If your left nostril is blocked, do not force the breathing. Try it after a few minutes.

4. Victorious breathing (Ujjayi breathing)

Ujjayi is often called the "victorious" or "sounding" breath. It involves constricting the back of the throat while breathing to create an "ah" sound—thus the "sounding" name.

Steps:

1. Sit comfortably with your back, neck, and head erect, and your hands on your lap. Close your eyes.
2. Use both nostrils for inhalation and exhalation. Keep your mouth closed.
3. Inhale with slowly constricting your throat partially in the back, partly closing the glottis, making an "ah" sound. The sound should come from the upper part of the throat and not from the nose. The indrawn air should strike the palette with soft, cool brushing effect. Inhale until the lungs feel full.
4. Hold your breath for four seconds.
5. Exhale slowly through both nostrils, constricting your throat again with the glottis partially open so the sound is heard again.
6. This is one round.
7. Practice five rounds for the first week. Then increase one round each week until you reach ten rounds.

Benefits:

- Ujjayi breathing massages the throat, nasal passages, and lungs, and strengthens them.
- It gives relief from sore throats, colds, allergies, and coughs.
- It helps to focus the mind and increases mindfulness.
- It generates heat in the body.

Caution:

Do not use force with the inhalation and exhalation.
Do not put too much pressure on your throat, only a slight pressure is needed.
If you have a cold or if you are coughing, do not practice this breathing exercise.

5. Bellows breathing (Bhastrika Pranayama)

Bhastrika Pranayama imitates a "bellows" (a device with an air bag that emits a stream of air when squeezed, for blowing at a fire to keep it going). This is a dynamic and energizing exercise.

Steps:

1. Sit comfortably in Easy pose or Lotus pose with your hands on your knees. Close your eyes.
2. Take a slow breath in.
3. Breathe out quickly and a little forcefully through the nose, but do not strain.
4. Immediately breathe in with a little force.
5. When you breathe in, your abdomen moves out and your diaphragm contracts. When you breathe out, your abdomen moves inward and the diaphragm relaxes.

6. The body should remain steady. Your shoulders should not move at all, only your lungs, abdomen, and diaphragm should move in and out. The movement of the stomach is like a bellows.

7. The air creates a sound as it moves in and out the nose. It should not be a loud sound. It comes from the nose and not from the throat.

8. Continue breathing, not too deep, in and out quickly for ten breaths. Then take a deep breath in and exhale slowly.

9. This is one round. Practice five rounds.

10. After practicing for a week, add one more round per week until you reach ten rounds.

Benefits:

- This Pranayama increases the flow of air and oxygen in the body. It refreshes the body and mind and gives an energy boost.
- The abdominal muscles, chest, and lungs get strengthened.
- It activates the liver, pancreas, spleen, and the entire digestive system.
- It increases the exchange of oxygen and carbon dioxide in the bloodstream.
- It stimulates the metabolic rate and flushes toxins out.
- It helps to burn fat and lose weight.
- This exercise gives a good massage to the respiratory system.

Caution:

Do not use force with the inhalation and exhalation. Excessive force can induce dizziness or lightheadedness.
Stop if you feel you are hyperventilating.

If you feel fatigued after the exercise, you are doing it too forcefully.

If you have high blood pressure, a hernia, or lung ailments, do not practice this exercise.

If you have migraine or any type of headache, do not practice this Pranayama during the headache. Practice it when you are free from pain.

Use caution when practicing this exercise at high altitudes, as the oxygen levels are low in the air.

6. Cooling breathing (Sheetali)

Steps:

1. Sit in a comfortable pose with your hands on your knees and close your eyes.
2. Open your mouth and roll your tongue in a U-shape. It can be a small curvature of the tongue. If that is not possible, keep the tongue flat with mouth slightly open.
3. Place your tongue between the lips with the tip of the tongue protruding slightly beyond your lips. Breathe in slowly and deeply through your tubular tongue. The air flows over the moist tongue. You will feel the coolness on your tongue and on the upper palette.
4. Close your mouth and exhale through your nose, using both nostrils.
5. This is one round. Practice ten rounds.
6. After practicing for a week, try to hold the breath after inhalation for four seconds and then exhale through the nose.

Benefits:

- The breath becomes cool and it makes the body temperature cool.

108

- It calms the mind, reduces mental tension, and lowers blood pressure and anxiety.
- It reduces anger and irritability.
- It decreases acidity in the stomach and improves digestion.
- It stimulates the parasympathetic nervous system and relaxes you.

Caution:

If you suffer from a cold, asthma, or bronchitis, avoid this breathing exercise.

Do not practice this breathing in a room where the temperature is very cold.

Do not force the breath. If you feel dizzy during the practice, stop.

7. Humming bee breathing (Bhramari breath)

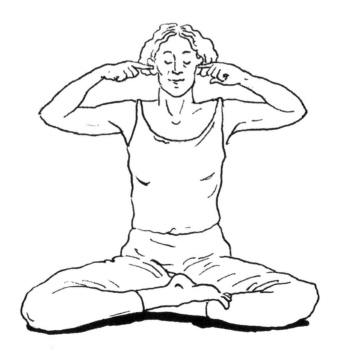

Steps:

1. Sit comfortably in Easy pose or Lotus pose. Close your eyes.
2. Inhale slowly and deeply through your nose.
3. Put your index finger into your ear, closing it. (Put right index finger into your right ear and left index finger into your left ear).
4. Exhale slowly and completely making a soft humming sound. Keep it low pitched and focus on the sound.
5. This is one round. Practice five rounds.
6. Lower your hands and open your eyes.

Benefits:

- Bhramari breathing relieves mental tension and stress and relaxes you.
- It reduces depression, anxiety, migraines, and hypertension.
- It improves the quality of sleep.
- This breathing helps if you have thyroid problems.
- It strengthens respiratory organs.

Caution:

Inhalation and exhalation should not be forced. It needs to be slow and smooth.

8 Yoga of Meditation (Dhyana Yoga)

Meditation has been practiced since antiquity and is a component of many religions. You do not have to be religious to practice meditation because the purpose of meditation is to calm the mind. Our mind is constantly jumping from one thought to another. It is restless all the time. It gets tired and does not function well and we get irritated and frustrated. The Yoga of Meditation gives us an opportunity to clear our mind and experience peace and self-control. The "mind-body" author and physician, Dr. Deepak Chopra says, "Meditation is not a way of making your mind quiet. It's a way of entering into the quiet that's already there, buried under the 50,000 thoughts the average person thinks every day." We simply need to be willing to encounter and explore our own mind. Meditation is a natural, simple, and effortless process. It is also a healing process. It is a stress reduction break, a refreshing break that you can give yourself wherever you are. Meditation is considered safe for all age groups. It is especially beneficial for older people since it reverses the effects of aging.

Actually, meditation is a built-in ability of the human body-mind system. It is something that our body knows how to do. If you set up the conditions and allow it, it will naturally go into a meditative state. It is a state when we give our permission to our brain, nervous system, and senses to do a tune up. It is our genetic heritage for our mind-body healing. It gives your system a profound rest, which is better than resting by lying down with your eyes closed, or even resting by deep sleep. Meditation also gives you an opportunity for self-observation and self-discovery.

An important aspect of the Yoga of Meditation is to witness our thoughts. Witnessing the thought process means to be able to observe the natural flow of the mind while not being disturbed or distracted. The more you can become a witness to these thoughts, the less control those thoughts have over you. It frees you from unnecessary thoughts and increases your freedom of choice. When we learn to ride a bike or drive a car, there is a learning process of how to focus on the task. Once we understand the process and the steps that are required, it becomes quite simple. Mind-observation is also a process, which is quite simple. As we practice it for a while, a better understanding of our own mind dawns upon us.

The fact that "I am not my thoughts" is one of the most fundamental and important of all principles of the science of Yoga. The thoughts that drift in our mind are good and bad, happy and sad, clear and clouded, but none of the thoughts are who we are. It is no longer a theory from some book, or the mere statement of a teacher. This kind of direct experience is the goal spoken of by the ancient yogis. The Yoga of Meditation gives us a direct experience. It is said that you should never just believe what you read or are told, but that you should also not reject these ideas either. Rather, we need to take the principles, reflect on them, do the practices, and find out for ourselves, whether they are true or not. Meditation gives us that unique experience of connecting to our core.

Newly published research indicates that the meditation technique activates our brain's natural "ground state." We usually have awareness of the three states: waking state, sleep state, and dream state. Each of these states has a certain brain pattern. The brain patterns of the meditative state are quite distinct from these three patterns. It means that our brain is capable of functioning on a new level. Actually, meditation is a "state" of mind and not a technique that we practice. We can achieve that state when we sit down and practice. In this state, we touch the essence that exists within us all. All of us have the ability to experience joy or bliss in this state. The Yoga of Meditation helps in achieving an emotional balance through detachment. Usually we are excessively attached to people, things, and outcomes. Meditation creates conditions where you are not affected by the happenings around you. This, in turn, creates a remarkable calmness and a positive outlook, which also has tremendous benefits on the health of the body and mind.

Ralph Waldo Emerson, the great philosopher and the man known as an American Transcendentalist, wrote, "Within man is the soul of the whole; the wise silence; the universal beauty, to which every part and particle is equally related, the eternal ONE. And this deep power in which we exist and whose beatitude is all accessible to us, is not only self-sufficing and perfect in every hour, but the act of seeing and the thing seen, the seer and the spectacle, the subject and the object, are one. We see the world piece by piece, as the sun, the moon, the animal, the tree; but the whole, of which these are shining parts, is the soul." Here Emerson describes a clear experience of that natural "ground state" of the brain!

Meditation uses the human ability of focused attention to begin the practice. The data on prehistoric times shows that even the older civilizations used repetitive, rhythmic chants to appease their Gods. The act of focusing our attention on a certain object or word or phrase makes our mind calm and other thoughts slowly subside. This gives us a process of clearing our mind. We need this clearing because the thoughts are entering our mind from all directions. It seems like we are bombarded by thoughts all the time. Some thoughts go away quickly and some thoughts linger. We like the pleasant lingering thoughts and we dwell on them, making them stay longer in our mind. Nevertheless, there are unpleasant lingering thoughts that we don't want to have, and yet they persist and make us miserable. The practice of meditation gives us the ability to go past, both pleasant and unpleasant thoughts and to see what is beyond. Our mind is bigger than the thoughts it contains. It is like the sky where we see some clouds. The clouds are like our thoughts, always coming and going, moving around, appearing and disappearing constantly.

The hectic pace of modern life is becoming more and more demanding. The more conveniences we have that are created by technological innovations, the more stress they are producing in our minds. We are dealing with too many things, too many people, and too much information. In addition, for us to handle, let alone digest all this, we feel we do not have enough time. We get tired and frustrated. Our mind becomes agitated and it stays in an agitated state. This creates many disturbances in the health of the body, which in turn disturbs the mind even more. It seems like we don't have any control over our life. We yearn for restfulness, for peace and quiet, for calmness and control over our own life. Some people think that if the body is calmed, everything will be all right. So they give the body caffeine, alcohol, tobacco, or drugs, which numb the body, giving temporary relief and creating enormously harmful side effects. However, the problems do not go away in this process; actually, they increase in many ways. Then we realize that we need something else to solve the problems. The Yoga of Meditation comes to help us at any stage of life, no matter what condition our body and mind is in. It lets you start wherever you are and allows you to go forward with many rewards on the way.

There have been many scientific studies done on meditation in the last thirty years. They include the effects of meditation on chronic pain, weight problems, stress, cardiovascular problems, digestive problems, insomnia, behavioral problems, anger, depression, and many more health disorders. The physiological and chemical changes resulting from meditation can be measured in the laboratory by testing blood levels of glucose, cholesterol, and other hormones, and also by administering EEGs, taking blood pressure readings, counting the pulse, and reading muscle-tension sensors. Amazingly, the conclusions of these studies indicate that meditation helps the patients in lowering the harmful biochemical levels in the body. Meditation promotes better sleep, better digestion, less pain, and overall better health. Research on the brain patterns of meditators indicate that their neural coordination associated with focus, memory, decision making, and learning is different than non-meditators' patterns. In regular meditators, they have found a higher level of melatonin than non-meditators. The neuroscientists involved in this research hypothesized in the past that regular meditation actually alters the way the brain is wired, and that these changes could be at the heart of claims that meditation can improve health and well-being. Now it can be seen with actual measurements. A few years ago, Dr. Rosenthal, a twenty-year medical researcher from the National Institute of Mental Health began to investigate other possible therapies to treat bipolar disorder. He selected the meditation technique. His preliminary findings show this program to be a fully safe adjunct to conventional therapies, and produces marked benefit for depressive patients.

On the physical level, the Yoga of Meditation helps each cell in the body to refresh, regenerate, and strengthen itself. As we sit down and practice meditation, the body is still, which helps all the systems—the nervous system, respiratory system, digestive system, circulatory system, and the rest of the systems. Sitting still with breathing slowly gives a good rest to all organs. As we practice a little longer, we go deep into the meditation and receive profound rest for our entire body internally. The internal rest is different from the external rest we give our body. In this restful state, as the breathing slows down, the heart beats at a slower rate, which decreases the load on the heart, the blood vessels relax and blood pressure decreases, the cortisol (the stress chemical) level goes down, and the exchange of oxygen and carbon dioxide becomes efficient. It makes our metabolism slow down so the digestion becomes better. The improved flow of air to the lungs helps breathing problems like asthma.

Meditation works on the body and the mind simultaneously. On the mental level, it improves learning ability, memory, and creativity. It helps to decrease anxiety, depression, irritability, and moodiness. It increases the subjective feeling of happiness and contentment. People with smoking, alcohol, and eating addictions who have been trained in meditation break their addictions with significantly lower relapse rates than those receiving standard therapies. Meditation sharpens the mind and brain so we can notice more details in any situation that might otherwise be missed. We know that paying attention to anything requires time and effort. Since we have a limited amount of both, we tend to overlook many things. In recent years, scientists have found that regular meditation practice made the areas of the brain bigger that are linked to attention and sensory perception. In meditation, we go to a state where our mind is not analyzing and judging anything so it is at its natural state. From that state, we receive better self-control and self-confidence.

A recent study on seniors, funded by NIH showed that meditation changed patterns of activation in the brain, shifting the focus of activity from the stress-promoting right frontal cortex to the left side, which is associated with a sense of well-being and positive emotion. In this 2004 study, the participating group meditated for only twenty minutes twice daily, resulting in stress reduction and lowering their blood pressure. [4] The effects of meditation on aging show that it slows aging.

Meditators look younger than their chronological age. Within all the research and studies, an important finding for the sixty-plus group is that the human brain remains moldable throughout life and new connections among the neurons (brain nerve cells) can constantly be grown. This process is enhanced with the practice of meditation. The effects of meditation go directly to the brain and directly to the cells. Imagine being able to rid yourself of health maladies without taking medications, and turning the clock back naturally! Meditation is the true anti-aging medicine because it activates our body's own natural anti-aging healing force. It is easy to do and with no cost, and is completely free from any side effects.

As we consider aging, our endocrine system is very important. Scientific studies have found out that meditation rejuvenates the pituitary gland, pineal gland, thyroid, and hypothalamus. It is effective for many ailments, including those associated with aging, such as change of life issues or menopause, Alzheimer's disease, arthritis, cardiovascular disease, and stroke, among others. A study of health insurance statistics on over two thousand people practicing meditation over a five-year period found that meditators consistently had less than half the hospitalization than did other groups with comparable age, gender, profession, and insurance terms. The difference between the meditation and non-meditation groups increased in older-age brackets. In addition, the meditators had fewer incidents of illness in seventeen medical treatment categories, including 87 percent less hospitalization for heart disease and 55 percent less for cancer. The meditators consistently had more than 50 percent fewer doctor visits than did other groups.

My father had a stroke after his retirement at age sixty-two. After his stroke, he could not do his asanas and go for his regular long walks. He said, "Now it is time to switch to another form of Yoga," and he decided to start doing meditation. He used to sit in his bed and meditate or lie down and meditate. It helped him to remain calm and peaceful with mental clarity. He kept on with his physical therapy and meditation until he passed away nine years later.

Types of Meditation

There are many types of meditations. We will see the four main types here. The details of these types are described later in this chapter. You can choose the type that best suits you and that you feel comfortable doing.

- **Breathing meditation**: The attention is focused on your breathing.
- **Sound meditation**: An effortless sound or word (a mantra) is repeated mentally with the natural rhythm of breathing
- **Guided meditation**: Listening to a CD or tape that gives you instructions on how to relax and let go of the tension in body and mind
- **Bead meditation**: Use of a rosary or japa-mala to repeat the name of God, a mantra, or a prayer

Preparation for meditation

The physical techniques of Yoga are the stepping stones to meditation. After you do the postures (asanas) and breathing exercises (pranayama), go ahead with the meditation. That is the proper flow of Yoga practice. If you are at your office or at the airport and want to do a short meditation, do slow and deep breathing for two minutes and then meditate. It is important not to use meditation as a replacement for your conventional care or as a reason to postpone seeing a doctor about a medical problem. Just add meditation to your routine and tell your physician that you are practicing it. It is important to find a meditation technique that fits you. It is like finding shoes that fit you well. If they don't, you will be uncomfortable. As you start practicing twenty minutes a day, you will notice how you feel during and after your practice. The effects of meditation last for the next twelve hours. That is the reason you need to practice twice a day to get full benefits for the whole day and night. Your practice will depend on your daily schedule. Sometimes we need to adjust our schedule to fit in two sessions of meditation practice. It is worth the adjustment. If one technique is not suited to you and you are not comfortable during the practice, you can try another technique of meditation. You will know the technique is right when you feel you are going deeper during the practice and feel calm afterward. It is a good idea to give yourself at least three months of practice to decide whether it works or not and then change to another form of meditation.

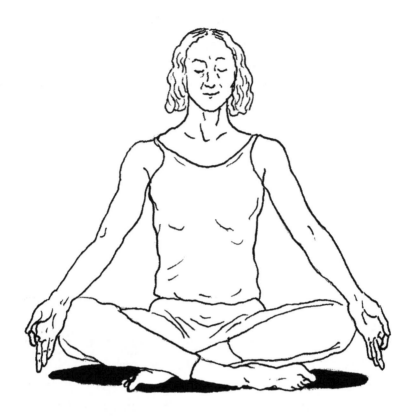

Start with choosing a quiet place and sit in a comfortable position, either in a chair with your back straight or on the floor on a small cushion or a folded towel. You can sit in Easy pose (Sukhasana) or Lotus pose (Padmasana). Your hands should be on your lap with palms downward, or you can place your hands on the knees with palms open. You should have all fingers open or join the thumb and forefinger. Keep your eyes closed during the practice. Breathe through your nose, with mouth closed.

What to expect during the practice

In the process of meditation, in the beginning, many thoughts enter and leave our mind. Focus on your breathing even when the thoughts are there; after a few minutes, the mind calms down, little by little. There are fewer thoughts, less feelings, the breathing slows down, the heart rate slows down, and the body relaxes more and more. You will remain alert and aware during the practice of twenty minutes. You will go into a deep relaxed state when all the functions in the body are at a different level of functioning—the brain wave patterns are in the alpha state and the nervous system is in a calm state. This is a new state. This is a natural state for the body-mind system for healing and rejuvenation.

During your practice, if you are able to "tune out" the world or the ticking of the clock in the room, even if just for a second, you are into the first stage of meditation. If you have a steady mantra repetition and are keeping hold of your mantra for a time, you are practicing meditation. You might experience this focused state for a few seconds in the beginning and after some practice, slowly, over a period of time, you will remain in that state longer.

After twenty minutes, we need to come out of this state very slowly; there should not be a quick getting up. The nervous system needs time to adjust from a deeper state to an awakening state. First, you need to stop focusing on breathing or on your mantra and stay relaxed for two or three minutes, and then open your eyes slowly; move the fingers, arms, and neck. Breathing will be back to the regular rate and then you can get up slowly. If you get up too quickly, it will be a shock to the nervous system and you might get a headache. The same is true if there is a phone near you that starts ringing suddenly or if there are other interruptions. You definitely need a quiet environment for twenty-five minutes. After your practice, if you look in the mirror, you will see your eyes are relaxed and your face is relaxed. You will know that the practice is working. Your own sense of peace, clarity, and joy will tell you what is happening to you. The peace you feel will spill over into your daily life and you will be able to handle anything that comes your way.

Some people get sleepy during the practice. In that case, you need to stop the practice slowly, giving yourself two to three minutes to come out of it and go to sleep immediately. Feeling sleepy during meditation indicates that your body needs sleep. Sometimes the flow of thoughts is so strong that it is hard to keep your focus on the breathing or on the mantra. At those times do not stop in the middle; continue the practice for twenty minutes. Your mind may be busy with thoughts but your body or some organs are getting the benefit of your practice.

1. Breathing meditation

Sit quietly, with your gaze downward, and slowly close your eyes. Inhale and exhale slowly and smoothly, allowing no jerks or irregularity to disturb the steady flow. Your chest and ribs should slightly expand while your shoulders remain motionless. Breathe evenly so your inhalations and exhalations are of the same duration. Be aware of your slow breathing. You will begin to feel the air flowing in your nostrils. Your mind will be calm, focused, clear, fully awake, and alert without being agitated. The thoughts in the mind will slowly disappear because your attention is on your breathing only and on nothing else. When your mind is in this state, it changes your physiology and centers you. This position is in between action and rest. It is awareness of yourself.

Think about it for a moment; you are breathing consciously. The process of breathing is both conscious and autonomic. In our sleep, we breathe automatically without any awareness of it. Breathing is a bridge between our conscious and subconscious mind. Practicing breathing meditation is one of the ways to bridge the gap between the conscious and subconscious mind. It integrates the mind so it can work as a whole toward your goals and beliefs rather than being pulled apart in several directions.

Breathing links us to everyone else. We all are breathing the same air that surrounds us. We all share this life-giving source, whether we are healthy or sick, rich or poor, from this country or that, whether happy or sad. We all constantly do this one thing, all our life. Now, doing it consciously is different because it increases our awareness as we do it. First, we become aware of our own self. We feel calmer inside; and this is a new feeling because we rarely feel the inside of us. This process automatically relaxes us. When the turbulence of distracting thoughts slowly subsides and our mind becomes quiet, a deep contentment and well-being arises from within. This is quite powerful, since we can see that we do not have to depend on any externals to feel peace. We get a warm peaceful feeling toward all. As we practice breathing meditation twice a day for twenty minutes, our mind gets used to this peace within and keeps that peace with us for the rest of the time.

The benefits of this meditation that we see right away are the calmness and joy in our mind. It gets into our relationships right away. People notice the change in you and comment on your happiness and joyfulness. It helps in personal relationships and in work relationships. Another benefit is that we can handle any situation without getting stressed or confused. Our abilities increase as we practice regularly.

2. Sound meditation (Mantra Meditation)

There are physical impurities in our organs and cells, which we can remove by Yoga exercises of asanas and a good diet. In our mind, there are impurities like fear, anger, greed, compulsiveness, and other negative emotions. They can be more damaging than the toxins in the body. Some of them are on a deeper level. The physical and mental exercises help a lot, but sometimes we need something more than that. It is not possible to purify the mind by consciously thinking about it. It seems that we are stuck with anger when we are angry, and we are stuck with fear when we are afraid. We need some way to get unstuck. The sound meditation or mantra meditation is a way to get unstuck. It works on many levels of our being—physical, mental, emotional, and spiritual levels. It gives us the ability to go beyond our conscious levels of understanding. Our mind transcends deeper and the effect of it is healing from the impurities of the mind. The mind heals itself. It happens slowly as we practice twice daily for twenty minutes. Initially, twenty minutes are needed for our mind to go deeper. Later on, this time can be increased slowly to thirty minutes.

The practice of sound meditation is done by sitting quietly in a chair with your back straight or on the floor in Easy pose or Lotus pose, with your eyes closed. Breathe slowly and smoothly through the nose. As you become aware of your inhaling and exhaling, say a word silently. This word can be the name of God or Goddess from your own spiritual tradition or a sacred phrase or the word "Om." You can use any peaceful word like serenity, tranquility, joy, or peace. There are certain beneficial vibrations to these words. The meaning of the word is not as important because the vibratory effects they produce when repeated verbally or silently are powerful. Repeat your word slowly and continuously with slow breathing. Keep your attention on this word and not on any other thoughts. If other thoughts arise, gently bring the focus back to your mantra. Practice this repeating either verbally or silently for ten minutes, at first. After ten minutes, stop saying the word and slowly open your eyes. Give yourself two to three minutes to come out of it and then get up. Slowly increase your practice to twenty minutes.

Yoga through sound meditation works remarkably to achieve harmony between mind and body. The word or mantra is in our mind, but there are other thoughts too. As we focus on our mantra, the other thoughts slowly subside, but they spring back again and again; and we go back to our mantra again. That is the process of this meditation. Every thought that comes to our mind has something attached to it, and that is some kind of emotion. As we focus on the mantra, the mind becomes peaceful because the mantra does not have anything attached to it. Our mind-body system likes this kind of peace. As we practice, our breathing slows down, our heart beats slower, the brain patterns go into alpha state, the blood vessels relax; all the processes in the body slow down and get a deeper rest. At this restful, relaxed state, healing takes place. It happens in the body and mind simultaneously. You are awake and aware during the practice. In this peaceful state, the mind is not clinging to anything; it is free. The old baggage is not weighing it down.

Sometimes in the beginning, too many thoughts come up to the surface and it seems that the meditation is not working, but you need to continue the practice because it is working on some other levels. Do not stop it in the middle; gently say the mantra and stay with it. Meditation is simply letting go and allowing yourself simply to be. Your mantra is your vehicle to go forward, as it makes its way, removing the obstacles. In the body, it removes the obstacles that are toxins and disorders. For example, many people say that if you have a mild headache and you practice mediation, the headache disappears. If you are taking medications for some health conditions, by all means continue with them, do not stop taking them. Just add meditation to your daily practice and the effects of this practice will become noticeable after a while. Meditation is a kind of medicine for the body and mind. It has no negative side effects.

We know that all matter—from the tiniest DNA strand in us to the largest of continents—is in a state of constant vibration, resulting in the emission of subtle sounds. The great teachers of ancient times did a lot of research and discovered that specific sounds energize specific portions of the brain. They used these sounds as mantras for meditation. The mantras act upon our bodies by reprogramming the vibrations of the cells and restoring them toward harmonious health conditions. The beauty of a mantra is that even a mechanical repetition gives you the benefits of its vibrations. Sound has enormous power; in fact, it has the power to create the entire universe. It is written that God originally manifested as sound. "In the beginning was the Word, and the Word was with God, and the Word was God" (John 1:1-2).

Transcendental Meditation™ was introduced by Maharishi Mahesh Yogi, and it is a form of silent mantra meditation where the practitioners receive a personal mantra. The Buddhist meditation practice uses the mantra "Om Mani Padme Hum." Some popular mantras are "Om or Aum" (the primordial sound or the sound of creation), "So-hum" (from breathing in sound "so" and breathing out sound "hum"), "Om Shreem" (goddess of abundance - Lakshmi), "Om Aaeem" (goddess of intelligence – Saraswati), "Peace Be Still," "Jesus," "Krishna," and "Rama." Some people repeat phrases from scriptures, such as "I can do all things through Christ who strengtheneth me," "The Lord is my Shepherd," "Om namah Shivay" (meaning I bow to Lord Shiva who is the God of transformation), or "Om Shanti, Shanti, Shanti" (Shanti means peace). These phrases and the phrases from all spiritual practices around the world are also powerful mantras. If repeated continuously for some time, they give you many benefits over anxiety and restlessness and heal you from many disorders, giving you self-control.

3. Guided Meditation

Guided meditations are very helpful for a specific area with which you need help. They are available on CDs or tapes, and you can listen to them any time. They usually are fifteen minutes to forty-five minutes long and they take your mind to the desired area of the body or mind. Listening to words spoken by someone has a very powerful effect on the mind. The suggestions that you hear go deep into the mind, stay there, and produce an amazing effect. They lead you by using words, step by step, to the desired result.

Guided meditation can be used to obtain peace of mind, enter a holy place and receive guidance, feel the presence of God, reflect on a concept or emotion, such as love or forgiveness, get freedom from addictions, heal the mind, heal a disease or disorder, surround yourself with love, relax the body and mind, sleep better, remove anger, gain understanding, increase your abilities and skills, create success and abundance in life, improve your relationships, become strong and healthy, lose weight, become friendly, manage your stress, or enhance your life.

The first step is to make your body relaxed. Since the body and mind are closely connected, by relaxing the body, the mind automatically starts to relax. It takes some time for the body to relax though. The guided meditation usually starts with slow and deep breathing and relaxing one part of the body at a time. Starting with toes, slowly you go to the feet, calves, knees, thighs, abdomen, back, chest, arms, neck, face, and head, and relax each. It is very important to go into the relaxed state in order to focus the mind on a specific area that needs help. The suggestions received in this state become powerful.

Some guided meditations include visualization. The imagery is effective because imagery is the most fundamental language of humans. When we recall events, we always see them in terms of pictures, sounds, images, joy, and pain, and hardly through words.

Our brain's visual cortex processes images and it has a strong connection with the autonomous nervous system. Scientific studies have shown that soothing, uplifting images actually slow the pulse, slow the heart rate, and lower blood pressure. It can help trigger the release of hormones such as endorphins, which make you feel good. Brain scans have shown that picturing something and actually experiencing something are very close as far as the brain waves are concerned. Stimulating the brain with imagery has a direct effect on the nervous system. If the words guide you to picture yourself sitting at the beach on a tropical island, your muscles will actually relax and your skin will feel warm when the warm rays of the sun are mentioned. Likewise, if you visualize recuperating quickly from your surgery, you are likely to heal faster.

Sometimes for some people, meditation on your own does not work. The mind cannot get the focus that is needed. The mind is either too agitated or it is restless. In this case, the guided meditation helps as it guides continuously so the mind does not go in many directions; it stays with the voice on the tape. That voice becomes the guide and the mind follows the instructions. It is a convenient and simple way to get the focus back.   Guided meditation is used in chronic pain management and pain relief. Pain is the message that something is wrong. Our mind perceives the pain but the mind also has the ability to manage it or control it or to reduce the intensity of it. When we improve our inner awareness and mindfulness, we can make mental and physical changes in ourselves. At first, we can identify the area where the pain is and then we can use imagery and see that area as a dark area in the body. Then we can bring the light of healing to that area and visualize the dark area slowly disappearing. Visualization has a powerful effect, as the body and mind are focused together. The words on the CD or tape can lead you in this process. If we repeat this process every night, before going to bed, it gets integrated into our system and produces desired results. In a small study, researchers at Pennsylvania State University in University Park,

PA, and Case Western Reserve University School of Medicine in Cleveland, OH, found that people who suffered from recurrent canker sores in their mouths significantly reduced the frequency of their outbreaks after they began visualizing that the sores were bathed in a soothing coating of white blood cells.

Many athletes use guided meditation and visualization to enhance their performance in sports. It is used in leadership training for effectiveness in public speaking, achieving goals, and for success in big undertakings. It is a powerful tool to create a healthy, happy, and optimistic view of life.

4. Bead Meditation

The use of a rosary or japa-mala is a practice of meditation in many religions around the world. It is the easiest and safest form of meditation and can be practiced by anyone at any time, and under any conditions. It is performed by repeating a prayer or mantra simultaneously with the rotation of a rosary or japa-mala. Using a rosary or a japa-mala for mantra meditation is very effective, as it provides an anchor to bring the mind back from wandering thoughts to the meditation. It is a tool and an anchor to keep your fingers on the beads and the mind on the prayer. The continuous movement of the fingers keeps the flow of repetition going. You can also keep a count of your prayers or mantras. In some traditions, there is a belief that when you do the count of 100,000, you get the desired result.

Hindu japa-malas

Japa means repetition of a mantra and mala means a string of beads or flowers, or any objects. Mala beads are generally made from different materials such as tulsi (basil) wood, sandalwood, rudraksh seeds, or crystals. Each type of material has certain properties that subtly affect the subconscious mind of the practitioner. The malas are made up of 108 beads, as the number

108 has spiritual significance. There are 108 energy lines at the heart that will be activated with this practice. In addition, there are 108 earthly desires that we want to overcome. The practice is started with the large bead, called the guru bead or meru bead.

During the practice of japa, concentration is most effectively centered when mala beads are held in the right hand. The left hand rests on the lap. Hold the beads in your right hand for about one minute. Let all of your energy flow into your hand and into the mala. Hold the guru bead, close your eyes and silently pray. Then start repeating the mantra by holding the mala near your lap and moving the beads by progressing the thumb and middle finger on to the next bead. If you wish to continue chanting upon returning to the guru bead, turn the beads in the opposite direction rather than crossing over the guru bead. Feel the sound vibration of the mantra continuing within you on a more and more subtle level. You can practice saying the mantra aloud or practice silently. You can keep your eyes open or closed. Some people go for a walk and practice this japa. If you are sick, you can do japa lying in your bed. It is especially helpful when you are restless or filled with fear.

Buddhist rosaries or malas

Buddhist malas come with 108 beads, fifty-four beads, and twenty-seven beads. At their base is the large guru or meru bead, which is the symbol of activity and movement. On the Buddhist rosary, the three beads directly above the base bead represent the Three Refuges: homage to the Buddha, homage to the Dharma, and homage to the Sangha.

A 108-bead Buddhist rosary is divided into six groups of eighteen beads, with a divider bead between each group. A fifty-four-bead mala has six groups of nine beads, with a divider between each group. A twenty-seven-bead mala has two groups of six beads and one group of fifteen beads, with two divider beads.

All divider beads in a rosary represent points of pause for silent meditation while holding the hands in prayer position.

In Japanese Buddhism, the beads are known as "juzu" and in Chinese Buddhism, they are known as "shu zhu"

Christian rosaries

The rosary may be used in prayers in many ways to mark the passage of particular prayers and to commemorate spiritual litany. To recite the rosary, hold the cross, make the sign of the cross and say the Apostle's Creed, say the Lord's Prayer on the large bead, three Hail Mary prayers on three small beads, Gloria (Glory be to the Father) prayer, ten Hail Mary prayers on each decade (a group of 10 beads) being terminated with the Gloria (Glory Be to the Father). Each decade is said in honor of some mystery, which is set apart for meditation during the recitation of the prayers. Proceed to the second mystery the same way, and so on.

The Apostle's Creed: "I believe in God, the Father Almighty, Creator of Heaven and earth; and in Jesus Christ, His only Son, Our Lord, Who was conceived by the Holy Ghost, born of the Virgin Mary, suffered under Pontius Pilate, was crucified; died, and was buried. He descended into Hell; the third day He arose again from the dead; He ascended into Heaven, sitteth at the right hand of God, the Father Almighty; from thence He shall come to judge the living and the dead. I believe in the Holy Spirit, the holy Catholic Church, the communion of saints, the forgiveness of sins, the resurrection of the body, and the life everlasting. Amen."

The Lord's Prayer: "Our Father, Who art in heaven, hallowed be Thy name; Thy kingdom come; Thy will be done on earth as it is in heaven. Give us this day our daily bread; and forgive us our trespasses as we forgive those who trespass against us; and lead us not into temptation, but deliver us from evil. Amen."

Hail Mary: "Hail Mary, full of grace. The Lord is with thee. Blessed art thou amongst women, and blessed is the fruit of thy womb, Jesus. Holy Mary, Mother of God, pray for us sinners, now and at the hour of our death, Amen."

Glory Be: "Glory be to the Father, and to the Son, and to the Holy Spirit, as it was in the beginning, is now, and ever shall be, world without end. Amen."

Muslim rosary

In Islam, a chaplet of ninety-nine beads, called "Tasbih," generally having a pendant with a special knot of richer material and a tassel, is used to recite the ninety-nine names of Allah. Often, a special bead is added called the iman or "leader," which stands for the inexpressible name of God. The prayer used is "Allahu Akbar" (Greatest is Allah). The beads are made of ivory, pearls, amber, rosewood, or olive wood.

Beads used by other cultures

Ancient cultures used sea shell beads or seeds for prayers. Native Americans use turquoise beads, clay beads, or wooden beads for meditation.

9 Yoga of Devotion (Bhakti Yoga)

Devotion is a very personal aspect of each individual. Devotion is an internal attitude of deep trust and love for the divine. We express it with our prayer, worship, or religious practice. The Sanskrit word for devotion is Bhakti. The word "devotion" implies focus on God and the devotee. Bhakti Yoga is a term that denotes the spiritual practice of fostering loving devotion ("bhakti") to a personal form of God. Our relationship to God is important to us. Bhakti Yoga is the practice of devotional disciplines, gratitude, reverence, surrender, worship, prayer, chanting, and singing, with the aim of awakening love in the heart and opening oneself to God's grace. Devotion is in our attitude, which means it is a matter of our heart. And our mind goes where our heart is. Devotion requires faith that comes from the heart, from the deeper part of us. With that faith, the negativity falls away. We all have heard of complete surrender to God or to a Higher Power for the joy of it. There are no requests, no desires, no pleasure-seeking intentions; it is just surrendering, without any attachments, which is the best state of mind. The devotees in the world know this state, and their minds function from that state. All practices of Yoga—postures, breathing, sense control, meditation—support devotion and are supported by Bhakti.

We are born and we deal with life in the form of people, things, events, actions, reactions, and duties. If we fix our mind on God and do all these things, we are devoted. Now, it is not easy to do it. Our mind goes after many things, constantly wandering from one object to another, seeking pleasure all the time, feeling many different emotions along the way. So how can we fix our mind on God? We can keep our mental focus on a deity or a symbol of God. That is a concrete object and not an abstract concept. Our mind can grasp a concrete object easily. Prayers and singing the hymns or devotional songs is a form of the Yoga of devotion. Some people maintain the focus by saying God's name and repeating it continuously for a certain time. They do it while doing their chores or while waiting for an appointment, or while cooking, or even when they are feeling anxious.

My maternal grandmother had an "acceptance with a smile" way toward all people and all events. I never saw her angry or upset at anyone. She was a great storyteller. I used to pester her for a story all the time and even though she suffered from asthma and would be coughing and wheezing, she would go on with her long stories. She told me the stories of ancient times and modern times, of religious and social issues, and of great heroes of the past. She did not have a formal education, but her intelligence and her wisdom was amazing. I was so impressed with her ways that once I asked her when I was eleven, "Aaji, when do you spend time learning all these things?" She said, "Oh, I just spend my time in practicing devotion to Goddess Lakshmi and that's all." I didn't know the meaning of devotion, so I thought it must be something very hard. Goddess Lakshmi is the goddess of wisdom and abundance. There is a famous temple of Lakshmi where my grandmother lived. The daily routine of my grandmother included an early morning walk to the temple, sitting in front of the deity, and praying there; after coming home, spending time in puja (the ritual of devotion to Lakshmi at home), chanting her name while doing her chores and while cooking, doing japa in the evening, and reading scriptures before going to bed. All day, her mind was fixed on her beloved goddess and it reflected the peace that came from devotion. Now I see what an amazing tool she used all her life!

Devotion also means service to God's creation. We see that some people are dedicated or devoted to a cause. It becomes so important to them that they forget everything else and keep on going. Dr. Albert Schweitzer, the great humanitarian, medical doctor, theologian, musician, writer, and missionary whose life was dedicated to his work in Africa, said, "As the sun makes ice melt, kindness causes misunderstanding, mistrust, and hostility to evaporate." He devoted all his energies to the hospital he established in Lambarene, French Equatorial Africa, where there was no doctor within five hundred miles. He performed eight hundred surgeries a year, even in his seventies. Half way through his eighties, he had been known to go seventy-two hours without sleep when one of his patients had been in danger. His caring for the world made him keep on working and writing—twenty-four major works of philosophy, religion, ethics, and a survey of world problems are to his credit.

Two important components of devotion are faith and love. All religions around the world speak about these two important aspects. Love is primarily self-giving—giving yourself to your beloved through feelings, thoughts, and actions. Devotion involves giving of yourself loyally and with deep affection. The heart has always been seen as the essence or center of a person. From the heart springs the love—for God and for His creation. This deep devotion makes a continuous flow of energy between God and the devotee and gives the devotee glimpses of superconscious awareness. The devotees can go beyond human limitations and experience higher consciousness, as we see in cases of great philosophers, poets, writers, and scientists. Many of us have some experiences of clarity for a few moments in our prayers. Devotion also creates peace and joyfulness in the heart, which also spreads to others.

My friend Lisa practiced Yoga postures, devotion, and japa with the Krishna mantra for many years. Last year, at age sixty-five she suddenly felt ill. The tests revealed that she had colon cancer, which was at a later stage and was inoperable. None of us could believe it, as we saw her as a very active, enthusiastic, caring, and strong person. Three of us, her friends, went to see her after we heard the sad news. We were crying and sobbing and couldn't comfort her. But she was in complete control and had all the spiritual wisdom to impart to us, with a smile. She said, "You know, every time the thought of cancer comes to my mind, I start my japa. The touch of each bead gives me strength. When I go to my eternal Home, I want to go with satisfaction for my life and with happiness." Her battle with cancer went on for four months. Actually, it wasn't a battle; it was intense devotion in the face of a difficulty. Her smile was always there, a barefoot walk in the backyard was a daily routine, resting in bed while using her japa mala was a constant practice. Her enthusiasm for small things never diminished; her love of life transformed into gratefulness and her prayers gave her strength and calmness. Her eighty-eight-year old mother came from Germany to see her; they spent two days praying together until Lisa passed away in complete peace. We all watched her during her last four months and realized something that she was showing us—the fear we all have of cancer or diseases or of dying has no control over us; we control whatever happens until the end!

Another way of devotion is to sing aloud God's name, in the form of hymns or devotional songs. It lifts the heart immediately and elevates the consciousness. It clears the mind and fills the environment with pure energy. Devotional singing originates in the heart and it is the joyous expression that wells up within the heart when the glory of God is remembered. Singing together with chanting, or "Kirtan," is a spiritual practice in India that literally translates as "celebrating, glorifying, and praising" God. It is not about artistic achievement or perfection, but rather about reaching a meditative state of mind. This practice creates an intense experience. In addition, when we repeat god's name, it gets recorded in our consciousness. After many repetitions, it creates a deep impression or a deep groove. This groove becomes more prominent than other grooves, like a groove of fear.

When we are devoted to something or committed to something passionately, we find more energy for it. It seems like more energy is generated inside of us. Moreover, time goes by too fast while we are engaged in it. How does it happen? Where does the extra energy come from? It comes from the attitude of devotion. What will drain our energy is the act of holding it back. The more you give and express the energy, the more will be generated. There is no need to force yourself to give, but you need to experience it.

The most effective devotion is a simple, direct prayer—just talking with God and then being still. This way shows us that by devotion and receptivity we can open ourselves to the reality of God and attract God's consciousness into our own. Love and devotion also can purify human nature and cleanse the mind and the emotional field. There can be no fear, hate, dislike, jealousy, envy, or prejudice in the loving heart. The truly blessed are the pure in heart, for they can perceive the reality of God.

10 Yoga for specific conditions

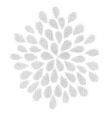

Yoga can become the "preferred medicine" that we all need in our health care system. It is a great tool for the hygiene for our body and mind. Yoga gives us much-needed nurturing, physically, mentally, emotionally, and spiritually. We need all four aspects of nourishing on a daily basis. The modern lifestyle creates an enormous number of sick people, and there is a huge cost to repair the sickness. Actually, the cure is not available. What is done is to find ways to merely numb the pain and numb the problem. Yoga practice goes to the root of the problem and corrects it over a period of time. After this correction occurs, we will be well connected to our own body and mind. Otherwise, we will remain divided as our mind says one thing, our body responds in another way, and our feelings go the third way. This fragmentation creates a lot of problems and pains. When we integrate these four aspects, we will have a feeling of well-being. Yoga practice brings these four aspects together.

Yoga is therapeutic and is a healing tool. Yoga therapy is widely used by people with health challenges and conditions. Medical research shows that Yoga therapy is among the most effective complementary therapies for several common ailments. We need both, the modern medicine and the ancient wisdom because they reinforce each other. The challenges we face may be an illness, a temporary condition like after-surgery recuperation, a chronic condition of pain, some weakness in parts of the body, or a disease. We need to remember not to stop the medications, but continue with them and start Yoga practice (consult your physician before you start any exercise program). We can choose certain postures or breathing exercises or meditation techniques that suit our individual needs.

Specific Yoga techniques that are helpful for various conditions are listed below by health condition, alphabetically. We will see why they are helpful and what changes take place when we practice certain postures or exercises. Each condition is followed by the suggested Yoga exercises that are helpful for that condition. The Yoga postures are described in Chapters 5 and 6. The breathing, meditation, and devotion Yoga are described in Chapters 7, 8, and 9. As mentioned in these chapters, gradually adding these postures to your basic Yoga practice will be more effective. After the practice of eight basic postures for two weeks, add one more posture, practice it for a week and then add more repetitions of it. You will see the benefits within a week or two. Then add another posture. This will increase the practice time every day, but it is worth spending this time. If one of the postures causes any discomfort, stop practicing it and try another one. Make sure there is no pain anywhere in the body during the postures. Be gentle with your body and remember to do the Relaxation pose (Shavasana) at the end of your practice. It integrates and balances the energies in the body.

Addictions

Suggested Yoga practice: Basic eight postures (in Chapter 5) for two weeks and then slowly add Sun Salutations, Alternate Nostril breathing, and Meditation.

A lot of bending and stretching in the Sun Salutations on a daily basis remove the toxins in the body and clears the channels. This exercise creates energy in the body. When the desire to drink or smoke arises, the Alternate Nostril breathing helps immediately because it balances the right and left hemisphere of the brain and gives control over the desire. The practice of daily meditation creates an inward focus, which in turn generates self-control.

Allergies

Suggested Yoga practice: Basic eight postures (in Chapter 5) for two weeks and then slowly add Sun Salutations, Ujjayi breathing, and Bellows breathing (Bhastrika).

The Sun Salutations give a lot of movement to the head, neck, throat, and lungs which loosens the phlegm and removes the stuffiness. The Pranayama (Ujjayi and Bhastrika breathing) regulates the channels of air in the body. It clears the nasal passages, sinuses, throat, and lungs. The pollens that cause allergies are carried away and eliminated from the body.

Alzheimer's disease

Suggested Yoga practice: Basic eight postures (in Chapter 5) for two weeks and then slowly add Sun Salutations, Relaxation posture (Shavasana), Alternate Nostril breathing, and Meditation.

The Sun Salutations stretch and massage the internal organs and the brain. Shavasana relaxes the body and mind while you are aware of the slow relaxation. The heart rate and breathing slows down and with it, and the blood pressure goes down. The Alternate Nostril breathing creates balance between the left and right hemisphere in the brain and improves communication between the two. Meditation creates a centered and grounded state and improves memory and recall.

Anemia

Suggested Yoga practice: Basic eight postures (in Chapter 5) for two weeks and then slowly add more repetitions of Easy posture and Mountain posture (Tadasana), and Right Nostril breathing.

The Easy Pose and Mountain Pose help with more blood circulation in the body. The Right Nostril breathing stimulates the digestive fire and improves the appetite. It also generates heat and energy in the body.

Anxiety

Suggested Yoga practice: Basic eight postures (in Chapter 5) for two weeks and then add Relaxation posture (Shavasana), Deep breathing, and meditation.

Shavasana relaxes the body and mind while you are aware of the slow relaxation. The heart rate and breathing slows down, and with it, the blood pressure goes down. The tenseness and stiffness melts away. During this whole process, you are aware of your breathing, and your focus is on your breathing. The anxiety-producing thoughts melt away in this pose.
In any tense situation, Deep breathing gives an instant relief from the tension-producing thoughts. Regular practice of meditation gives you the ability to remain calm and anchored in any situation. It also gives you self-control from overwhelming thoughts in any circumstance.

Arthritis

Suggested Yoga practice: Basic eight postures (in Chapter 5) for two weeks and then slowly add Forward Bend (Padahastasana), Chair posture (Utkatasana), Triangle pose (Trikonasana), Spinal Twist (Matsyendrasana), Cooling Breath (Sheetali Pranayama), and Chanting (Japa).

All joints in the body need lubrication and movement. The slow and controlled movement of joints is helpful for arthritic patients. Doing the Forward Bend and Chair pose slowly as far as you can go and staying in the pose for ten seconds helps to strengthen the joints. The triangle pose and spinal twist are helpful for the entire joint system in the body. In these poses, the blood circulation improves and flexibility is gained. In the beginning, there may seem to be more pain while doing the poses, but after slowly continuing the poses, the pain diminishes. The cooling breath helps the cooling of inflamed and painful joints. Chanting aloud or just listening to the sounds of Chanting helps the arthritic pain because of the healing vibrations of sound.

Asthma

Suggested Yoga practice: Basic eight postures (in Chapter 5) for two weeks and then slowly add Bow posture (Dhanurasana), Cobra posture (Bhujangasana), Shoulder Stand (Sarvangasana), Plow posture (Halasana), Downward Facing Dog (Adho mukhasana), Alternate Nostril breathing (Nadi shodhana), and Bellows breathing (Bhastrika).

These Yoga poses increase the air circulation in lungs and in sinuses, creating easy airflow. They also stretch the torso, chest area, throat and Trachea (windpipe), making them more flexible. The Alternate Nostril breathing allows the air to flow smoothly. It clears the blockages and strengthens the lungs. The shortness of breath and wheezing is replaced by deep breathing. The Bellows breathing exercises the entire respiratory system with rapid and short breaths. The continuous diaphragm movement clears the blockages.

Back problems

Suggested Yoga practice: Basic eight postures (in Chapter 5) for two weeks and then slowly add Lotus posture (Padmasana), Forward Bend (Padahastasana), Cat posture (Marjariasana), Spinal Twist (Matsyendrasana), Triangle posture (Trikonasana), Bow posture (Dhanurasana), and Child's Pose (Balasana).

The stretch your back receives during these postures helps reduce the back pain and makes the back stronger. Triangle pose works the hips, and the hips have a strong influence on the spine and the back. The spinal twist provides good stretching for the back.

Cancer

Suggested Yoga practice: Alternate Nostril breathing (Nadi shodhana), Meditation, and Chanting (Japa)

The Alternate Nostril breathing creates balance between the left and right hemisphere in the brain and improves communication between the two. It eases the pain in the body. The regular practice of meditation generates peacefulness, balance, healing, and a grounded feeling. It gives rise to the feeling of self-control. Chanting creates certain vibrations in the body that generates healing energy.

Carpal Tunnel Syndrome

Suggested Yoga practice: Basic eight postures (in Chapter 5) for two weeks and then slowly add Cobra posture (Bhujangasana), Downward Dog posture (Adhomukhasana), Mountain pose (Tadasana), and Prayer pose (both palms joining together, in front of your chest).

Carpal Tunnel syndrome is a condition that can cause pain, tingling, numbness, and weakness in the fingers, thumb, and wrist. It may be felt as pain all the way from the hand into the shoulder. It is a potentially debilitating nerve disorder of the hand, usually caused by repetitive motion, like typing. These postures strengthen the arms, wrists, and shoulders. They allow the hands and fingers to stretch and relax, causing better circulation.

Cholesterol (elevated)

Suggested Yoga practice: Basic eight postures (in Chapter 5) for two weeks and then slowly add Sun Salutations, Shoulder Stand (Sarvangasana), Cobra posture (Bujangasana), Spinal Twist (Matsyendrasana), Triangle posture (Trikonasana), Bellows breathing (Bhastrika pranayama), and Meditation.

The Sun Salutations stretch and massage the internal organs. It helps the fat to be effectively metabolized. The Shoulder Stand, Cobra pose, Triangle pose, and Spinal Twist reduce fat in the blood, increasing the level of HDL (high-density lipoprotein - good cholesterol). The Bellows breathing helps the digestive tract and metabolism in the body. It reduces waste build up in the blood, which in turn reduces undesirable cholesterol. Meditation reduces stress hormones, which in turn lowers cholesterol.

Colds

Suggested Yoga practice: Basic eight postures (in Chapter 5) for two weeks and then slowly add Sun Salutations, Alternate Nostril breathing (Nadi shodhana pranayama), and Bellows breathing (Bhastrika).

The Sun Salutations help to unclog stuffiness in the chest, nasal cavities, and in sinuses. The Pranayama breathing—Alternate Nostril breathing and Bellows breathing—makes the breath flow easily and it removes the chest congestion.

Colitis

Suggested Yoga practice: Basic eight postures (in Chapter 5) for two weeks and then slowly add Leg raise (Urdhva Prasarita Padasana), Locust posture (Shalabhasana), Side-to-side roll with knees to chest (Pavanmuktasana), and Bellows breathing (Bhastrika).

The colon area gets massaged in these postures and blood circulation increases. The movement of this area strengthens the colon. The Bellows breathing gives an in-and-out movement to the digestive system and the colon. It soothes the irritation in the walls of the colon.

Constipation

Suggested Yoga practice: Basic eight postures (in Chapter 5) for two weeks and then slowly add Sun Salutations, Leg raise (Urdhva Prasarita Padasana), Side-to-side roll with knees to chest (Pavanmuktasana), Cobra pose (Bhujangasana), and Bellows breathing (Bhastrika).

The Sun Salutations give an overall exercise to the digestive system and reset the balance in the tract. The Leg raise, Side-to-side roll with knees to chest pose, and cobra posture provide gentle pressure to the lower abdomen and relieves stagnation in the colon. The Bellows breathing provides quick movements of the stomach and digestive tract. It enables regular bowel movements.

Cough

Suggested Yoga practice: Victorious breathing (Ujjayi breathing) and Alternate Nostril breathing (Nadi shodhana)

These Pranayama breathing practices clear the nasal passages, sinuses, and congestion in the chest. They reduce coughing and sore throat. They massage the throat, lungs, and sinuses and strengthen them.

Depression

Suggested Yoga practice: Basic eight postures (in Chapter 5) for two weeks and then slowly add Sun Salutations, Shoulder stand (Sarvangasana), Plow posture (Halasana), Alternate Nostril breathing (Nadi shodhana), Right Nostril breathing (Surya bheda), Meditation, and Chanting (Japa).

The Sun Salutations generate heat and energy in the body, which removes the depressed state in the body and mind. It supplies more oxygen to all parts of the body. The postures of Shoulder stand and Plough pose reverse the effect of gravity and allow more blood flow to the brain. The Alternate Nostril breathing creates balance between the left and right hemisphere in the brain and improves communication between the two. The

Right Nostril breathing creates heat and energy in the body. The regular practice of Meditation generates peacefulness, balance, and a grounded feeling. It gives rise to the feeling of self-control. Chanting creates certain vibrations in the body that generates positive energy.

Diabetes

Suggested Yoga practice: Basic eight postures (in Chapter 5) for two weeks and then slowly add Sun Salutations, Locust posture (Shalabhasana), Sitting with Forward Bend posture (Paschimottanasana), Leg raise (Urdhva Prasarita Padasana), Lying twist (Jathara Parivatasana), Knees to chest (Pavanmuktasana), Bridge pose (Setu Bandhasana), Cobra pose (Bhujangasana), Alternate Nostril breathing (Nadi Shodhana), Humming bee breathing (Bhramari pranayama), and Meditation.

The Sun Salutations create energy in all the systems in the body and eliminate toxins. This vigorous exercise improves insulin administration in the body. The Locust pose, Sitting with Forward Bend posture, Leg raise, Lying twist, Knees to chest, the Bridge pose, and Cobra posture give an internal stretching to the liver, pancreas, and all the abdominal organs. Insulin production and distribution is regulated by these exercises.

Alternate Nostril breathing creates balance between the left and right hemisphere in the brain and improves communication between the two. The Humming bee breathing creates sound vibrations that are beneficial to all glands in the body. Meditation practice helps the endocrine glands through relaxation of the sympathetic nervous system. The glucose balance and digestion process get restored.

Digestive disorders (acidity, heavy stomach, indigestion, acid refluxes, gas, stomach pain, bad breath, diarrhea, Irritable Bowel Syndrome - IBS)

Suggested Yoga practice: Basic eight postures (in Chapter 5) for two weeks and then slowly add Sun Salutations, Leg raise (Urdhva Prasarita Padasana), Side-to-side roll with knees to chest (Pavanmuktasana), Cobra pose (Bhujangasana), Bow pose (Dhanurasana), Warrior1 and 2 postures (Virabhadrasana 1 and 2), Spinal twist (Matsyendrasana), Lying twist (Jathara Parivatasana), Relaxation pose (Shavasana), and Bellows breathing (Bhastrika).

The Sun Salutations give an overall exercise to the digestive system and reset the balance in the tract. The Leg raise, Knees to chest pose, Warrior1 and 2, and Cobra postures provide gentle pressure to the lower abdomen and relieves the stagnation in the small intestine and the colon. The Lying twist gives abdominal circulation. The Bow pose increases gastrointestinal circulation and reduces acid. These poses cause better food absorption and assimilation. The spinal twist stimulates the pancreas, liver, spleen, kidneys, stomach, and ascending and descending colon. The Relaxation pose calms down the digestive process and relaxes the abdominal organs.

The Bellows breathing provides quick movements of the stomach and digestive tract. It enables regular bowel movements.

Eye problems (conjunctivitis, inflammation, irritation, burning sensation, redness)

Suggested Yoga practice: Basic eight postures (in Chapter 5) for two weeks and then slowly add Cobra posture (Bhujangasana), Relaxation pose (Shavasana), and the Sun salutations.

The Sun Salutations and Cobra pose help the head, neck, and eyes move upward and downward. It helps blood circulation in the eyes. The Relaxation pose with eyes closed give complete rest to the eyes.

Fatigue

Suggested Yoga practice: Basic eight postures (in Chapter 5) for two weeks and then slowly add Lotus posture (Padmasana) or Easy pose (Sukhasana), Alternate Nostril breathing (Nadi shodhana), and Right Nostril breathing (Surya bheda).

Sitting in Easy pose or Lotus pose and breathing slowly resets the balance in the body and the mind. The relaxation pose relieves the tension in the body and generates strength. Alternate Nostril breathing creates balance between the left and the right hemisphere of the brain. Right Nostril breathing generates energy in the body.

Headaches (migraines, tension headaches, strain headaches)

Suggested Yoga practice: Basic eight postures (in Chapter 5) for two weeks and then slowly add more practice of Relaxation pose (Shavasana), Child pose (Balasana), Alternate Nostril breathing (Nadi shodhana), and Meditation.

The Relaxation pose and Child pose with eyes closed give complete rest to the body and mind and relieve tension in the head and forehead.

Alternate Nostril breathing creates balance between the left and the right hemisphere of the brain and removes stress. More oxygen reaches the brain and reduces the pain. A regular practice of Meditation creates calmness, slows down the heart rate, and relaxes the blood vessels in the head, reducing the pressure.

Heart problems

Suggested Yoga practice: Basic eight postures (in Chapter 5) for two weeks and then slowly add Sun salutations, Sitting on heels (Vajrasana), Forward Bend (Padahastasana), Cobra posture (Bhujangasana), Relaxation pose (Shavasana), Victorious breathing (Ujjayi breathing), and Meditation.

The Sun Salutations create better blood circulation in the entire body and strengthen the heart. More oxygen reaches all the organs and cells. The Forward Bend, Cobra pose, and Sitting on heels stretches the middle part of the body, heart muscles, and chest muscles. The relaxation pose slows the heart rate and relaxes the heart muscles. Victorious breathing contracts and expands the chest muscles, increasing the blood and air circulation. In deep meditation, the heart rate slows down and the heart remains in relaxed state.

In 1998, Dr. Ornish published a study in the *American Journal of Cardiology*, stating that 80 percent of the 194 patients in the experimental group were able to avoid bypass or angioplasty by adhering to lifestyle changes, including Yoga.

Hearing loss, ringing in the ear (Tinnitus)

Suggested Yoga practice: Basic eight postures (in Chapter 5) for two weeks and then slowly add Cobra posture (Bhujangasana), Cat posture (Marjariasana), Shoulder stand (Sarvangasana), Humming Bee breathing (Bhramari breathing) and Alternate Nostril breathing (Nadi shodhana).

The Cobra posture, Cat posture, and Shoulder stand stretch the neck and ears. The contracting and expanding of these areas create better circulation and strengthens the damaged nerves that cause problems. A regular Yoga practice increases GABA levels in the body. GABA (Gamma-Amino-Butyric Acid) is a brain neurotransmitter that inhibits electrical activity and reduces Tinnitus. The Alternate Nostril breathing balances the nerve centers in the brain. The Humming bee breathing generates sound vibrations that have a healing effect to the nerve endings in the ear.

Hemorrhoids

Suggested Yoga practice: Basic eight postures (in Chapter 5) for two weeks and then slowly add Fish posture (Matsyasana), Shoulder stand (Sarvangasana), Bridge posture (Setu bandhasana), and Child pose (Balasana).

The Fish pose, Shoulder stand, and Bridge pose lift the pelvic area and the colon area. These poses create more circulation in these areas, making them stronger. The Child pose stretches the pelvic area in the other direction. The combination of these poses reduces pain and inflammation.

Hypertension (high blood pressure)

Suggested Yoga practice: Basic eight postures (in Chapter 5) for two weeks and then slowly add Lotus posture (Padmasana) or Easy posture (Sukhasana), Cat posture (Marjariasana), Sitting with Forward bend posture (Paschimottanasana), and Relaxation posture (Shavasana). Practice Cooling breath (Sheetali pranayama), Alternate Nostril breathing (Nadi shodhana), and Meditation.

The Lotus or Easy pose keeps the body straight with heart rate slowing and creates relaxation in blood vessels, arteries, and veins. In the Cat pose, the contraction and expansion of chest gives a gentle massage to the heart. The kidneys become stressed from hypertension; sitting with Forward Bend posture (Paschimottanasana), the kidneys get strengthened. The Relaxation pose makes breathing to slow down and gives profound rest and calmness to the body and mind. The practice of Pranayama with Alternate Nostril breathing and Cooling breath creates a quick slow-down of all body functions.

A regular practice of Meditation creates peacefulness in the body and mind. The tension and stress melt away when the heart rate slows down. The blood vessels relax, blood pressure drops, and the mind-body system functions effectively.

Hypoglycemia (low blood sugar)

Suggested Yoga practice: Basic eight postures (in Chapter 5) for two weeks and then slowly add Locust posture (Shalabhasana), Fish posture (Matsyasana), and Alternate Nostril breathing (Nadi shodhana).

The Locust pose and Fish pose stimulate and strengthen the pancreas and kidneys. These poses prevent hypoglycemic symptoms of light-headedness, weakness, tremor, nervousness, rapid heartbeats, and nausea. Alternate Nostril breathing creates balance and calmness and provides more oxygen to all organs.

Impotence

Suggested Yoga practice: Basic eight postures (in Chapter 5) for two weeks and then slowly add Sitting on heels (Vasjrasana), Bow posture (Dhanurasana), Sun Salutations, Shoulder stand (Sarvangasana), Alternate Nostril breathing, and Meditation.

Sitting on heels and Bow pose provide some pressure to the pubic area and stimulate the area with more blood circulation. The Sun Salutations generate heat and energy in the entire body.

The shoulder stand creates rejuvenation of the glands. It has a marked effect on the pituitary, thyroid, adrenal, and sex glands. This produces a feeling of well-being, prevents premature aging, and extends sexual virility well into old age. Alternate nostril breathing creates balance and calmness and provides more oxygen to all organs. A regular meditation practice generates more self-confidence and self-control.

Insomnia

Suggested Yoga practice: Basic eight postures (in Chapter 5) for two weeks and then slowly add Sun Salutations, more time in Relaxation pose (Shavasana), Left Nostril breathing (Moon breathing), and Meditation.

The Sun Salutations in the morning or afternoon create an overall energy in the entire body. It helps to induce good sleep at night. The Relaxation pose helps to let go of all the tension, and then it is easy to fall asleep. Melatonin is produced by the pineal gland and released mainly at night during sleep. The Sun Salutation activity has been shown to increase production of melatonin. Melatonin is also a natural immune enhancer. The left nostril breathing activates the parasympathetic nervous system, which counteracts the effects of stress. It calms you down with slower heartbeats and relaxes the body so it is easy to fall asleep.

Kidney problems

Suggested Yoga practice: Basic eight postures (in Chapter 5) for two weeks and then slowly add Lotus posture (Padmasana), Easy pose (Sukhasana), Auspicious posture (Bhadrasana), Locust posture (Shalabhasana), Lying twist (Jathara Parivatasana), Fish posture (Matsyasana), Sitting with forward bend posture

(Paschimottanasana), Bow posture (Dhanurasana), and Bellows breathing (Bhastrika).

The Lotus pose, Easy pose, and Auspicious pose stretch the connective tissues of the outer thighs and buttocks and stimulate the kidneys. The Locust pose, Lying twist, Forward Bend, Fish pose, and Bow pose exercise, stimulate the kidneys, and increase circulation. The Bellows breathing, with quick movements to the kidneys, liver, and abdominal organs, creates more blood circulation. It creates better regulation of the secretions of the organs.

Menopause problems (hot flashes, irritability, and nervousness)

Suggested Yoga practice: Basic eight postures (in Chapter 5) for two weeks and then slowly add Sun Salutations, Auspicious posture (Bhadrasana), Lotus posture (Padmasana), Locust posture (Shalabhasana), Bow pose (Dhanurasana), Spinal twist (Matsyendrasana), Leg raise (Urdhva Prasarita Padasana), Knees to chest (Pavanmuktasana), Shoulder stand (Sarvangasana), Alternate Nostril breathing (Nadi shodhana), and Meditation.

The Sun Salutations raise the energy level and remove toxins from the body. The Auspicious pose stretches the pelvic area with more circulation. The Locust pose and Bow pose strengthen the lower abdominal area. The Spinal twist creates a good stretch for the back and stomach area. The Locust pose, the Leg raise, and Knees to chest pose stretch the legs and thighs, creating more circulation. The Shoulder stand massages the thyroid gland, pineal gland, and pituitary gland, and reduces facial wrinkles. It produces a natural "facelift." By doing the inverted postures for a few minutes each day, we can reverse the effect of gravity. The

155

Alternate Nostril breathing balances the left and right hemispheres of the brain and stimulates the glands, thereby creating hormone balance. A regular Meditation practice generates calmness, peace, and energy in the body and mind. It removes the imbalances, which are responsible for menopause problems. It restores natural well-being for the body-mind system.

Muscle cramps and spasms

Suggested Yoga practice: Basic eight postures (in Chapter 5) for two weeks and then slowly add Sun Salutations, Mountain posture (Tadasana), Sitting on heels (Vajrasana), Auspicious posture (Bhadrasana), Downward facing dog (Adhomukhasana), Triangle posture (Trikonasana), and Victorious breathing (Ujjayi breathing).

Muscles get tight and achy because of inactivity, tension, and stress. The Sun Salutations help by stretching and loosening all muscles in the body. The Mountain pose (Tadasana), Sitting on heels (Vajrasana), the Auspicious pose (Bhadrasana), and Downward facing dog (Adho Mukhasana) stimulate circulation in the body, and stiff muscles get relaxed and stretched. Then the toxins are carried away. The Triangle pose strengthens the hamstrings, thighs, leg, and arm muscles. Victorious breathing helps the chest, throat, and abdominal muscles.

Obesity

Suggested Yoga practice: Basic eight postures (in Chapter 5) for two weeks and then slowly add Cat posture (Marjariasana), Cobra posture (Bhujangasana), Fish posture (Matsyasana), Bellows breathing (Bhastrika pranayama), and Right Nostril breathing (Surya bheda pranayama).

The Cat, Cobra, and Fish poses give a good stretch to the middle part of the body where fat tends to accumulate. The Bellows breathing increases the rate at which the body burns off fat. The Right Nostril breathing generates heat and energy in the body, which is useful in burning calories. With normal aging, people tend to develop abdominal obesity. High levels of intra-abdominal fat has been found to be predictive of heart attack risk and is also linked to high cholesterol, high blood pressure, and high triglycerides. There is a strong association between increased waist circumference, insulin insensitivity, and type-2 diabetes. Yoga practice seems to weaken this link. It also keeps a steady level of DHEA (dehydroepiandrosterone - a steroid hormone that slows or reverses the aging process).

Osteoporosis

Suggested Yoga practice: Basic eight postures (in Chapter 5) for two weeks and then slowly add Mountain posture (Tadasana), Warrior1 and 2 postures (Virabhadrasana 1 and 2), and Alternate Nostril breathing (Nadi shodhana).

The standing poses—mountain pose and warrior poses—provide gentle stretching and strengthening for the body. Bending poses should be avoided.

Alternate Nostril breathing restores balance in bones and muscles.

Prostate problems

Suggested Yoga practice: Basic eight postures (in Chapter 5) for two weeks and then slowly add Lotus posture (Padmasana), Bow posture (Dhanurasana), Locust posture (Shalabhasana),

Shoulder stand (Sarvangasana), Spinal twist (Matsyendrasana), and Downward facing dog (Adhomukhasana).

The Bow and Locust posture stimulate the prostate gland and strengthen it. The shoulder stand inverts the flow of bodily fluids and gives relief to the organs. The spinal twist affects the entire pelvic region, which increases circulation. The Downward facing dog pose stretches the pelvic area. These poses stretch the whole body; stretching various glands results in increased efficiency of the endocrine system.

Smoking

Suggested Yoga practice: Basic eight postures (in Chapter 5) for two weeks and then slowly add Sun Salutations, Shoulder stand (Sarvangasana), Bow posture (Dhanurasana), Alternate Nostril breathing (Nadi Shodhana), and Meditation.

The Sun Salutations on a daily basis remove the toxins in the body and clear the channels. The inverted pose of Shoulder stand helps with circulation in the body and the Bow pose stretches the chest and lungs. When the desire to smoke arises, Alternate Nostril breathing helps immediately because it balances the right and left hemisphere of the brain and gives control over the desire. It stops nervousness and quiets the mind. The practice of daily Meditation creates an inward focus, which in turn generates self-control and stronger will power.

Stress

Suggested Yoga practice: Basic eight postures (in Chapter 5) for two weeks and then slowly add Sun Salutations, Shoulder stand (Sarvangasana), Spinal twist (Matsyendrasana), Bow posture (Dhanurasana), Victorious breathing (Ujjayi pranayama), Cooling breath (Sheetali), and Meditation.

The Sun Salutations create heat, vitality, and energy in the body, which helps to deal with stressful situations. The Shoulder stand, Spinal twist, and Bow pose stretch the body, resulting in increased circulation. They also create hormonal balance in the body. Victorious breathing and Cooling breath create calmness and reduce physical and mental stress. Feelings of insecurity, frustration, and nervousness slowly disappear from the mind.

Meditation gets the focus out of bothersome and irritable things and creates stillness. In that stillness, one can rise above the stress.

Urinary incontinence (bladder problems)

Suggested Yoga practice: Basic eight postures (in Chapter 5) for two weeks and then slowly add Sitting on heels (Vajrasana), Forward Bend posture (Paschimottanasana), Leg raise (Urdhva Prasarita Padasana), Bow posture (Dhanurasana), Plow posture (Halasana), Spinal twist (Matsyendrasana), and Alternate nostril breathing (Nadi shodhana).

Sitting on heels, the Leg raise, and the Forward Bend posture stretch the pelvic area and stimulate the functioning of the urinary organs. The inverted poses of the Plow and Bow postures create a reverse effect of the gravitational flow, and strengthen the urinary system. The Spinal twist stimulates the pancreas, liver, spleen, kidneys, bladder, stomach, and ascending and descending colon. The Alternate Nostril breathing restores the balance in the organs and brain.

Varicose veins

Suggested Yoga practice: Basic eight postures (in Chapter 5) for two weeks and then slowly add Shoulder stand (Sarvangasana) and Plow posture (Halasana).

The inverted poses of Shoulder stand and Plow are helpful for the enlargement and discoloration of veins. In these postures, the blood flows from the legs toward the heart, which is the opposite of the normal blood flow from the heart to the legs. This kind of flow relieves pressure, removes blood clots, and removes toxins.

Yoga postures for after surgery

Suggested Yoga practice: Gentle practice of standing posture – Mountain pose (Tadasana), Alternate Nostril breathing (Nadi shodhana pranayama), Cooling breath (sheetali pranayama), and Meditation.

Follow the advice of your physician after surgery regarding any exercise. Start with a gentle practice of the Mountain pose. It will strengthen the legs and upper body. Some stretching while lying down on your back is helpful in the recovery process because it improves circulation in the body.

The Pranayama practice of alternate nostril breathing creates balance in the right and left hemispheres of the brain and regulates the recovery process. The Cooling breath calms you down and provides a stable state. Meditation creates focus in the brain, which is useful for a quick recovery. Meditation can be done in a seated position or lying down on your back.

Yoga postures for other health conditions (not mentioned above)

For any health condition, practicing some form of Yoga postures is helpful. The practice depends upon every individual condition and the limitations of each person. The basic eight poses are the starting point. If you practice just the basic poses and do not add any other postures, you still will get the benefits. The key is the regularity of the practice. Spending just twenty minutes each day with Yoga practice goes a long way toward better health.

Yoga postures for individuals with disabilities

Chair Yoga: Mountain posture in seated position, Alternate Nostril breathing (Nadi shodhana pranayama), Cooling breath (Sheetali pranayama), and Meditation.

In addition to the Mountain pose exercise, you can do neck bending, neck rotations, arm stretching, arm rotations, shoulder rolls, and leg stretching while seated.

The Pranayama practice of Alternate Nostril breathing creates balance in the right and left hemispheres of the brain and regulates body functions. The Cooling breath calms you down and provides a stable state. Meditation creates focus in the brain, which is useful for self-confidence. Meditation can be done in a seated position or lying down on your back.

11 Yoga as a Lifestyle

The great American philosopher Ralph Waldo Emerson once observed, "Our health is our number one wealth!" Many of us have experienced a state of good health, balance, and the feeling of well-being. We also have experienced a state of imbalance or illness and weakness. The well-being consists of physical well-being first and then mental, emotional, and spiritual well-being. The science of Yoga gives us a way toward that well-being we want all the time. The steps for our well-being start with the practice of Yoga. The sister science of Yoga is called "Ayurveda" or science of life. It recommends the daily routines, diet, exercise, breathing, meditation, and a way of life for our well-being. Yoga practice does not take time from our daily routine; it gives us quality time. Making time for Yoga practice is time spent in honoring ourselves and dedicating some time for our nurturing. It is time spent in serving our own self. It is a part of serving others because we have more energy to give to others when we are energized with Yoga.

The science of Yoga includes eight areas according to the great sage Patanjali in his "Yogasutras" (the threads of Yoga). They are called eight limbs (Ashtanga) of Yoga.

- The first limb is Yama (restrictions) – no harming, no lies (truthfulness), no stealing, no craving on sensual level, and no unnecessary desires.
- The second is Niyama (observances) – cleanliness, contentment, austerity, study of scriptures, and devotion to God.
- The third is Asana – postures for making the body strong, healthy, and flexible.
- The fourth is Pranayama – breath control (for calming the body and mind).
- The fifth is Pratyahara – restraining of the senses from objects (non-attachment).
- The sixth is Dharana (concentration) – fixing the mind on one object or on the name of God or on a phrase.
- The seventh is Dhyana (meditation) – effortless concentration on the name of God or a phrase without other thoughts.
- The eighth is Samadhi – the state from ordinary consciousness to super consciousness.

In the previous chapters, we saw how to practice the third limb of Yoga, the practice of Asanas. Then we saw the fourth limb, the practice of Pranayama or breathing methods. The fifth limb of Yoga, Pratyahara, is the practice of self-control. The mind and body are attached to pleasure-giving objects and try to seek pleasure all the time, and that creates problems many times. The practice of controlling the senses gives us power over our destructive habits. The sixth and seventh limbs of Yoga, Dharana and Dhyana, consist of focusing and concentrating on the name of God or a phrase.

The first two limbs of Yoga give us the "do not" and "do" part of life. They are not meant to take any joy out of our life or serve in an authoritarian way; they simply make the practice of Yoga and one's well being easier to achieve.

The "do not" part, Yama, consists of the following:

o   Do not harm anyone by thoughts, speech, and actions. Avoid being unkind to anyone.
o   Do not lie, but be truthful. Do not speak bluntly to people about their shortcomings.
o   Do not steal. Get the things you need by proper means.
o   Do not have cravings on a sensual level. Keep the senses under control. Do not let the senses control you. Do not overuse your sexual energy.
o   Do not have excessive and unnecessary desires in life.

The "do" part, Niyama, consists of the following:

o   Practice cleanliness for your body, your house, and your surroundings. Next, keep your mind and heart clean.
o   Practice contentment or satisfaction and gratefulness for the people and things in your life.
o   Practice endurance, tolerance and purity. Make a commitment to do your Yoga practice regularly.
o   Keep your mind on spiritual ways, with studying scriptures (of your own religion).
o   Practice devotion and surrendering to God.

The eighth limb of Yoga is Samadhi, which is a state we reach when we are in deep meditation. It can occur for a few seconds when we are not aware of the passage of time or anything else. We are completely absorbed in meditation. This is a rare state and needs a lot of practice in deep meditation. However, a few glimpses of it make us want to reach it again and experience the joy of it. The great teachers describe this joy as "bliss," which is way beyond ordinary joy. The eight limbs of Yoga give us the way of life that is conducive to our well-being. When we keep these ways in mind and practice them on a daily basis, we will automatically make right choices. That is the beauty of Yoga and also the power of it!

Thinking

Our everyday thoughts determine the outcome of our life. In our everyday life, we consciously need to say "no" to our negative tendencies and impulses. But before we do that, we need to recognize those negative thoughts and tendencies in us. The practice of Yoga gives us better health; more oxygen to our brain and body; and a calm, alert, and peaceful mind, so our thinking goes toward better choices, and we acquire the ability to recognize the negative tendencies in ourselves.

The next step is to say "no" to those destructive tendencies in our thoughts, speech, and actions. Obsessive and unwanted thoughts disturb the peace of mind and create chaos and confusion in the mind. With that, the body gets into a chaotic mode with health problems. The question arises on how to keep our thoughts in control. It seems that the thoughts control our mind. But that is not true.

We have the ability to control our thoughts. It can be done with deep breathing. When we focus on our breathing as we inhale and exhale, our mind gets engaged in this process and other thoughts stop disturbing us. That is the reason breathing meditation or any meditation works when you practice it every day. It gives a profound rest to the restless mind and at the same time, it gives complete rest to the body. We acquire calmness and peace with this practice. This peace permeates the body, brain, and mind for many hours.

The reason for practicing meditation twice a day, once in the morning and once in the evening, is that we need to recharge the mind-body system on a regular basis so we retain the peace for twenty-four hours a day. Our thought patterns change as we keep on practicing, and they become more positive, more logical, more peaceful, and more powerful. It becomes easier to change the old harmful thought patterns into new beneficial thought patterns.

Medical researchers have found that brain waves become more coherent with the practice of meditation. It means we attain the ability to solve our problems in a better way with a positive outcome, without getting disturbed by them. As the mind becomes peaceful, the body responds with better health and more energy. This translates into more creativity and loving relationships. That is what we want for the rest of our lives!

Fresh air and sunlight

Our well-being depends on getting some fresh air every day and practicing deep breathing. After you get up early, give yourself half an hour of time, sit in the morning sun, and practice deep breathing. It will fill you with joyous energy. Or, facing the sun, do a meditation; it will connect you to the core of your spirit. Or go for a walk or a run. You will inhale more oxygen and you'll get sun on your body. What could be more invigorating than this? The Vitamin D you're getting in the morning sun has greater value than being in the sun later in the day. Sunlight generates negative ions. And negative ions purify air. In nature, negative ions are generated by processes such as sunlight, waves from the ocean, and from waterfalls. A morning walk in the sun or on a beach always leaves you feeling refreshed. Studies at Columbia University have shown that atmospheres charged with negative ions relieve hay fever and asthma symptoms, seasonal depression, fatigue, and headaches, and improve brain function and alertness.

One of the major benefits of sunlight is that it supplies Vitamin D, which not only promotes the absorption of calcium in the body but also transfers calcium across the cell membranes.

This, in turn, provides strength to the bones, as well as contributes to a healthy nervous system by increasing the production of endorphins and serotonin in the brain. Another significant benefit of sunlight is that it helps in the prevention of infections resulting from bacteria, molds, and viruses. The health benefits of sunlight include the enhancement of the immune system by increasing the count of white blood cells, as well as gamma globulin, which is beneficial in warding off viruses and germs and enhancing the capacity of red blood cells in carrying oxygen. About ten minutes of the sun on our face and body is adequate each day or at least four days a week. Overexposure to the sun can result in health problems such as melanoma/skin cancer or wrinkles. Remember that artificial light can never substitute for the real rays and the life-giving power from the sun.

Sleep

A good, restful eight hours of sleep is essential for our well-being. Sleep is the time when the body is able to rest, repair, and heal itself. We need to allow the body to have this precious time every night. The mind and emotions also become balanced during our sleep. The stress of the day melts away and we get rejuvenated. Recent research is suggesting that when we are asleep at night, our brain is actually performing specific tasks that process what we have experienced during the day. It sorts out our experiences and saves them for later retrieval. Think about the millions of bits of information we process each day. Some of our experiences, or the memory of them, need to be reinforced, and some need to be pruned. An important memory needs to have special channels opened for easy recall. A good night's sleep allows us to have memory recall of specific information when we need it. It is scientifically proven that a poor night's sleep affects our cognitive processes and our ability to have good memory.

We consciously need to remove the habits that come in the way of good sleep. These habits include worrying, excessive thinking about our problems by going round and round with the same thoughts, drinking stimulants throughout the day, eating too much beyond our ability to digest properly, getting stuck in destructive thoughts like anger and hatred, dwelling on past events, imagining future events, excessive attachment to some people, attachment to the outcome of our efforts, and thinking about only what is lacking. An important step when we lie down in bed is to let go of everything, pray to God, and relax physically, mentally, and emotionally.

My friend Wendy confided to me once that she tries all this but the thoughts just keep coming and keep her awake at night. And she feels tired all day the next day. She asked, "Is there a way to stop unwanted thoughts?" The spiritual teachers tell us that it takes a powerful thought to stop other thoughts. So the powerful thought can be a thought of God, the name of God, or a word or phrase or mantra in your own belief system. If you repeat this word for a few minutes with your eyes closed, it removes other thoughts, and the mind gets calmer, relaxed, and free. A free mind gets to sleep quickly.

Diet

The science of Yoga recommends eating the foods that increase the prana or life force. Eating right is really important, as our entire life depends on it. High-quality, balanced meals eaten in small quantities on a three-meals-a-day-plan is the best plan for our health. The science of Yoga recommends all six tastes— sweet, sour, salty, bitter, astringent, and pungent—in our diet every day. These six tastes create chemical balance in all the systems in the body. Eating fresh, organic, freshly cooked food provides nourishment to the body and mind. Good nutrition treats our whole body, from our organs to our cell level and then to our DNA level! It repairs the damage done by stress, age, illness, and pollution! This is a very effective protection, from macro to micro levels! All we need to do is to say no to junk food and processed food, and put the right food in our mouth.

The science of Yoga recommends whole grains, fresh vegetables and fruits, nuts, a lot of fiber, some dairy products (milk and yogurt), less fat, less sugar, and plenty of water on a daily basis. Fresh fruits and vegetables have the highest life force. Ice cold drinks and food are not recommended because they cause problems in the digestive system.

Eggs and meat are not recommended in Yoga diet because they are not considered pure foods. If you are used to having them in your diet, try to have them in very small quantities.

Yoga places great emphasis on eating slowly. If you eat fast or too quickly while doing something else, the food does not get digested properly. Our digestion converts food into energy-producing nutrients that support and sustain our body and brain. Poor digestion can lead to gas, a heavy feeling, and a build-up of digestive impurities.

Good digestion begins with a balanced appetite. Some people have no appetite, some cannot fully taste their food, and some people never feel satisfied. When a meal is prepared or selected carefully and really savored and enjoyed, it helps the body to prepare for proper digestion and assimilation. The three important aspects of food are digestion, assimilation, and elimination. We need to pay attention to all these aspects. Good balanced meals and good exercise everyday automatically give us good elimination.

Cleaning your plate whether you are hungry or not is not a good idea; honoring your digestive system is a better idea. After a meal, your stomach should be 50 percent full with food, 25 percent full with water, and the remaining 25 percent should be empty, with room for digestion to take place. Yoga places emphasis on "mitahara" or moderate diet. After practicing Yoga for two months, and learning about moderate diet, Martha in my meditation group was hooked on the idea of mitahara. She just started eating less of everything. At first, she didn't feel satisfied after her meals, so she started adding more vegetables and fruits in her plate. That did the trick. She lost forty pounds in six months. She has continued with this new habit and is feeling fit and healthy at age sixty-four. She no longer likes the too-full feeling and she is not stressed about her weight. Her meditation practice helped her to shift her focus from her weight to her connection to her inner self. On the emotional level, first, she gained self-acceptance, and that made it possible for her to observe her eating habits. It is an internal process that is much more effective than just dieting.

You not only are what you eat, but you act like what you eat. Food affects our mood, behavior, and relationships. If you eat foods that create a sense of well-being for you, your relationships will be happier too. The Yoga diet helps us to achieve our ideal weight and maintain it. It helps us to have physical, mental, and emotional balance. It is a proven and trusted path to better health in later years and for longevity.

Fluid intake

Drinking plenty of fluids prevents dehydration, which is the cause of many disorders in later years. Our bodies need eight cups or sixty-four ounces of water each day. The plain water helps digestion, keeps the Electrolyte balances in the body, and prevents memory problems. If you are on medications, you will need more water. Fluids like fruit juice or milk are additional to the water requirement. Some the other fluids like sodas, coffee, and alcoholic beverages do not have any positive value and need to be avoided or consumed at a minimum level.

Removal of toxins

We do not like to think of our bodies as active toxic waste sites, but something like that happens. Toxins build up in our body faster than it can purify them. The pollution from air and water, food chemicals and preservatives, emotional stress, and poorly digested foods create deposits of toxins in the body. If these deposits do not get eliminated, they become breeding grounds for harmful bacteria, disease, and sickness. It is similar to oil in a car that becomes thick and filled with sludge while ruining the parts of the engine. According to Yoga, cleansing the body of toxins is essential for creating good health.

It is essential to have elimination or daily bowel movements. Some deposits in the colon are deeply plastered to the walls of colon and we cannot get rid of them by regular bowel movements. If you experience symptoms of low energy, fatigue, weight gain, or some of the other diseases, even if you exercise and eat right, the cause of this is the toxins in the body. We need a colon cleanse or colon irrigation with water (colonics) once a year. The practice of colon cleanses dates back to ancient India and Greece. In the United States, it was used in the 1920s, but it lost support and was stopped. Recently, it has become available in many cities due its effectiveness. A fasting with fruit juices for two days and a colonic will remove a lot of toxins from the body and positive effects on the health are immediate. There are different ways of doing a colon cleanse, from a five-day liquid fast with daily colonics to a longer program. A colon cleanse is not recommended if you have ulcerative colitis, Crohn's disease, hemorrhoids, recent bowel surgery, kidney disease, or heart disease.

For blocked nasal passages, colds, sinuses, allergies, head-aches, and ear-nose-throat problems, the use of a Neti pot is rec-ommended. The Neti pot comes from the Yoga/Ayurveda tra-dition and has been around for thousands of years. It is a small ceramic or stainless steel pot with a small spout for the flow. It can flush out the nasal cavities by using gravity to draw the flow of water. The water needs to be made into saline solution by adding one-fourth teaspoon of salt into one cup slightly warm filtered water.

Fill the Neti pot with this solution and stand near the sink with your head tilted 45 degrees and slightly forward. Keep the mouth slightly open and pour the water into the top nostril slowly by inserting the tip of the spout in that nostril. The water will flow through the nasal cavity and into the other nostril, and out through the other nostril, in a continuous stream. Use half the water and switch to the other nostril. It clears the nasal pas-sages and sinuses very quickly and gets rid of harmful bacteria and pollen deposits. The use of a Neti pot is recommended once or twice a week.

Our sweat contains more toxins than urine. Research stud-ies have been done to confirm that the most effective way to get rid of toxins and heavy metals from the body is to sweat them out. The use of heat for removal of poisons from the body dates back to ancient times when saunas were created. After our daily exercise, we need to allow our body to sweat. We need to take a shower afterward to wash away the sweat and the toxins from the skin. Also, we need to remember to drink plenty of water in order to avoid dehydration.

Moderation and balance

Yoga emphasizes moderation in everything in our daily life. The food we consume need not be too much or too little. Many of us have had the experience of eating too much and feeling bloated with heaviness in the stomach and an uneasy feeling for the rest of the day. On the other hand, in the name of dieting, consuming too little food, we feel depleted of energy and feel tired. The body does not get nourished in both these cases. The quantity of food should be balanced and appropriate for energy and strength. Yoga does not recommend fasting unless it is for a colon cleanse.

Moderation in our sleep is important for our well-being. Sleep should not be too much or too little. Many of us have the experience of getting too much sleep; we wake up heavy-headed and groggy. If we get too little sleep, we feel tired and uneasy and lose focus on our work. Sleep needs to be appropriate, from six to eight hours.

There needs to be moderation in doing our work. Working too much does not mean we are more productive. The right number of hours spent in working with the right amount of time in relaxation gives us a better balance for our health and for our well-being.

We hear from medical practitioners to have moderation in alcohol, limiting to just one drink a day; but Yoga says that there is no need of alcohol. It is harmful to the body and mind. Also smoking, drugs, too many medications, and unnecessary medications need to be avoided.

There needs to be moderation in buying unnecessary things, spending too much on vacations, seeing too many movies, and spending too much time watching TV, or on the internet. There is a place for these things in life but balance is the first thing we need to consider.

Having some quiet time being alone each day is a basic requirement of humans, from our childhood till the end. This alone time gives us a chance to focus on our self, seeing our needs, wants, goals, and feelings. It is a daily check-up, which results in keeping ourselves nourished, fit, and healthy.

Relationships

Our relationships are very important to us. Basically, we are related to the earth, air, water, and food for our survival. Then we are related to people in our life, and they include our own family members, relatives, friends, co-workers, our community, animals, our country, and our world. We consciously need to have a harmonious relationship with these elements. As soon as any problem arises in any of these elements, we suffer a great deal. When these elements work nicely in our life, we feel the joy of life.

In order to keep ourselves happy, we need to take the responsibility on our own shoulders to make these elements work in loving, productive, and harmonious ways. It means saying "no" to many harmful things like hate, prejudice, anger, insult, ignorance, stress, judging others, blaming, faultfinding, meanness and hurting others in our thoughts, speech, and actions. When these enter our mind, we need to replace them with understanding, thoughtfulness, helpfulness, compassion, kindness, goodness, gentleness, forgiving attitude, self-control, and love. This requires a shift in our thought patterns and actions, which happens gradually as we practice Yoga.

We know the joy of having a good conversation with someone. It is uplifting and leaves us with more energy. What happens in a good encounter? Both parties feel they expressed themselves well; they feel they were heard well, acknowledged well, were encouraged by the other, were admired by the other, and received some help as well as understanding and love from the other. That is the kind of relationship we want at home, at work, with our friends, and with the world.

The most important relationship we have is the one with our own self. In order to check that relationship, see how you feel when you are alone. If you are at peace, comfortable with your own company, and at ease with yourself, then you have a positive relationship with yourself. If you feel you have to be with someone who will love you or you have to be doing something, or you need some stimulant to feel better or you feel lonely, then your relationship with your own self needs some work.

We tend to find love from outside, from someone, as if it is a material thing that you receive from someone. With Yoga practice, we feel the love inside of us. When we feel it, we can easily give it to others. And when we give it, as a result, we receive more from others. Love without any strings attached is something that always gets reciprocated in some form.

Productivity

We feel satisfied when we are productive. We are productive when we do housework, cook, clean, shop for groceries, send a cheerful note to a friend, do volunteer work, give advice when asked, rake leaves in the yard, write an article, listen to a friend, do a crossword puzzle, visit a sick relative, practice Yoga, go for a walk, play with a child, create an oil painting, and in many more ways. Going to work and spending eight hours at the workplace is not the only way of being productive. Many people do not feel productive after they retire from work. However, work-place related work is only one area of life. We can remain productive all our lives, no matter what our age. If we remain engaged in life, engaged with people, our energy gets circulated and it reflects in our health. Seniors, with their experience, knowledge, and skills can add more value to society in a way they feel comfortable. It does not mean they need to spend many hours doing something; just a few hours each week would be advantageous to them and the society in which they live.

Some people decide not to think about their age and instead think about their goals and aspirations. Grandma Moses, the famous American painter who started painting in her seventies, lived to 101 years of age and remained active right until the end. She said, "Painting's not important. The important thing is keeping busy." John Glenn resumed his career as an astronaut at the age of seventy-seven when he rode in the space shuttle Discovery. He famously said, "Too many people, when they get old, think that they have to live by the calendar," What an age buster! In some societies, the elderly are respected because of their wisdom and understanding and their opinions are considered valuable. We see that successful aging is largely determined not by genetic inheritance, as commonly believed, but by individual lifestyle choices in diet, exercise, pursuit of mental challenges, positive thinking, self-confidence, and involvement with other people. This is a very optimistic outlook. We gain it when we practice Yoga in some form, either asanas or breathing exercises or meditation. It is no wonder that the life span increases when we practice Yoga.

Relaxation and laughter

In order to relax, we need to throw away non-essential numbers like our age and weight! We need to enjoy simple things in life and laugh a lot. Life offers many things every day to laugh about. A study done on a group of volunteers at Loma Linda University showed that a good laugh increased participants' beta-endorphins, which are natural stress-relievers and pain-reducers.[5] Also, laughter is good for your heart; it improves your heart rate, lung function, and blood oxygen level. It can lower your blood pressure and reduce the risk of cardiovascular disease. There are groups in some cities that practice "Laughter Yoga" together.

Laughter eases muscle tension and strengthens the immune system by increasing the production of infection-fighting antibodies. It can instantly lift your mood and you will feel refreshed. Laughter helps in your relationships. When you laugh with someone, you create a bond and become more open to interactions with that person. Laughter is very contagious and it strengthens human connections. Keep cheerful people around. The only person who is with you all your life is yourself. So keep yourself cheerful too.

Another important thing to remember is to surround yourself with what you love and what inspires you. Tell the people in your life that you love them at every opportunity. Let go of the regrets, sadness, guilt, and blame from the past. There will be times when you have to endure some events and grieve. Taking it as a part of life and moving on with our life is the best way. Our home is our refuge so we need to keep it clean and cheerful. Getting the sun in the house reduces molds, dampness, and bacteria in the house.

Keep learning about something you like. When we learn something new at any age, new brain patterns form and grow. Our brains have the capability for growing neuron-connections all our life. That is the kind of growth we want all our life. It keeps us engaged with life and gives us something to look forward to each day. What could be better than learning about Yoga if you have not tried it yet?

Contentment

Yoga puts a great deal of emphasis on contentment. Being happy with what you have, being grateful for what you have in life, creates joy. The tendency of our mind is to focus on what we do not have and then go after those things with all our energies. Not feeling satisfied with what you have creates more desires and more greed for things to acquire. More things do not mean more joy. There is a notion that if you spend a lot of money on something, it will give you more satisfaction. But real satisfaction comes without spending anything. It is generated inside of you; it is free and it fills you to the fullest. Real satisfaction can be found in simple things, like - a nourishing meal, a good time with a friend, a joyful conversation with a family member, helping someone, reading a good book, a walk in the woods, relaxing in the sun, watching the stars at night, admiring the beauty of flowers, watching children play, painting a picture, or spending time in your hobby.

In the "Yogasutras," the great Yoga teacher Patanjali says, "Good health, strength, beauty, and charm are possible rewards of yogic practice." This is true all our life and well into our later years!

12 Personal evolution

All life forms have an impulse to evolve. The intellect, the magnitude of which separates humans from all other animals, developed slowly over four million years or more of human development. The awareness or consciousness of humans is expanding continuously, right from birth and throughout all our lives. The practice of Yoga helps the evolution of human consciousness. It is a journey, and as we consciously or knowingly expand our awareness, we feel this new energy in our lives. The practice of Yoga consists of welcoming this new energy and new joy into our lives.

Buddha said, "We are shaped by our thoughts; we become what we think. When the mind is pure, joy follows like a shadow that never leaves." Human beings are evolving in their thoughts. Evolution means a change, a change in thoughts and circumstances. The human cerebral cortex has grown in size over the last few millennia. The capabilities of our neurons are increasing; the neurons have the capability of higher spiritual experiences. People normally change very slowly. Usually it requires a crisis to radically change a person. The crisis can be personal like a health problem, bereavement, pain, or dissatisfaction, and it can be socio-political like a war or a natural disaster. The history of humankind clearly shows that each person has some immature and harmful attitudes and beliefs. They get replaced by more harmonious ones when the person goes through a crisis.

Another way a person consciously goes for a change is when the person suddenly realizes his or her mortality. As we look at our life, we realize that we are hanging on to some ineffective thoughts and actions. And then we resolve to change ourselves. The change is not easy since our habits are deeply ingrained in us. We consciously need to let go of the old thoughts and acquire new thought patterns. Meditation is a scientific technique that enables us to do it. It has been around for thousands of years, in every religion, in every part of the world. A steady practice reveals to us the power that is within us. We value our own free will and we take responsibility for our life. That is how we go forward with our evolution.

As we evolve and change, our mind expands. This expansion gives us a new joy. We get the ability to see and listen to the subtle levels of our body and mind. Our internal perception gives us a great deal of help. Recently, I had my echocardiogram and I saw my heart beating on the screen. I realized how it is beating continuously for many years without rest, with the blood pumping and valves opening and closing, constantly at work. I thought, "What an amazing organ!" Sometimes we need a concrete visual image to believe it. I felt great respect for my heart and then felt love for it. We may think of our love as coming from the heart but I think it originates from the mind. The mind is the ultimate perceiver. Then I thought about the other organs, how they are working constantly too. As our perception of our body and mind changes, we feel better physically, mentally, and emotionally, so we delve into it even more. We feel like we are explorers in a new realm. Our perceptions, understanding, and connectedness grow as we practice Yoga.

The great scientist Albert Einstein wrote, "A human being is part of the whole called by us the Universe, a part limited in time and space. We experience ourselves, our thoughts and feelings as something separate from the rest. It is a kind of optical delusion of consciousness. This delusion is a kind of prison for us, restricting us to our personal desires and affection for a few persons nearest to us. Our task must be to free ourselves from the prison by widening our circle of compassion to embrace all living creatures and the whole of nature in its beauty. The true value of a human being is determined by the measure and the sense in which they have obtained liberation from the self."

When our awareness expands, more things in life make sense because our perspective changes. Then our response to life becomes more positive. Instead of reacting to situations, we respond in a better way. We spend less time on things that do not matter much and have more time for meaningful activities. The solutions to problems become obvious and quick. We experience less resistance because there is less fear and more clarity. As a result of this, we experience a new freedom. It gives us an opportunity to be in harmony with the process of life. We remain open to new possibilities that life may bring our way. As we look around, we see the opportunities to extend our hand, our time, and our love.

Letting go of the things we previously held on to—the outcome of everything, people in our life, our self-image, and material things—becomes easier. These factors created a sense of dependence. When we let go of these factors, we feel the freedom. The free mind is a powerful mind.

The best thing we can do for the world is to focus on our own personal growth and transformation. Once we do that, we automatically act from that level. Rather than reacting to someone quickly and impulsively, we will give ourselves space and opportunity to think before we act. That space translates into expanded awareness. In there we find inner resources— self-confidence, self-reliance, faith, good health, and abilities! And they get stronger as we practice Yoga. In our daily life, when we are faced with challenges like an illness or a difficult relationship, it helps to remember that within us are our inner resources. Even if we forget to use them, they are still there. They give us clarity, ease, and an anchored and stable state.

Creativity is a remarkable force that forever changes our life. Each of us has a unique type of intelligence and unique type of creativity. As we expand our awareness, we need to diversify our interests and find some creative work. Giving ourselves more diverse and rich experiences will bring more vitality to our life. We usually stick to our comfortable zone in order to create certainty and structure to our life, but finding new areas of growth gives us a deep satisfaction and a sense of adventure. We do not need to find time for this, we need to make time to go out, give love, be with people, explore nature and new places, know different cultures, and see the world. That is where the greatest fulfillment is found. It can be for the self or for the community, or for the world at large.

The human body is a vehicle that carries the mind and spirit. We need to keep this vehicle fit and strong all our life. The ancient seers and yogis gained expanded awareness by the practice of Yoga. They transcended the limitations of mind. In the process, their intuition became very powerful. They researched and developed many branches of Yoga for people of different temperaments. These additional types of Yoga practices include:

- Karma Yoga – practice of selfless action and service with non-attachment
- Jnana Yoga – practice of using intellect and knowledge
- Raj Yoga – a path to unity through meditation and renunciation

- Kundalini Yoga – practice of using psychic nerve centers (chakras)
- Yantra Yoga – practice of using vision and forms
- Tantra Yoga – specific techniques for using and controlling body-energies
- Mudras – hand and finger gestures used for healing and balancing energies in the body
- Bandhas (locks) – are used for binding back or capturing the dissipative energies in the body

In the Vedic literature, as well as in the Bhagavad-Gita, all forms of Yoga are described. The Bhagavad-Gita (the song of God) consists of the knowledge that Lord Krishna imparted to his warrior friend Arjuna on the battlefield. Arjuna was in confusion and in dilemma about life and his actions in life, about what is right and what is wrong, which path to take, how to stay balanced under difficult conditions, and how to have faith. Arjuna could not leave everything behind, go to the forest, and meditate all the time. He needed some guidance in staying connected to the world and doing his best. That is what each of us need in life. In a beautiful verse, Lord Krishna says, "God is seated in each person's heart. With full faith, when you ask for guidance, it will come from your heart." The Bhagavad-Gita gives importance to the power that is within us.

A great yogi once said, "The world is the great gymnasium where we come to make ourselves strong." In our life, we are always going from less strength to greater strength, from less knowledge to more knowledge, from less well-being to a better well-being, from less love to greater love, from small acts of kindness to big acts of kindness and from less understanding to a better understanding. We feel better when we are going in this direction. And even if we start going in a wrong direction, we can still start from that point and go forward. That is the natural flow of our evolution. Being in this world, we get plenty of opportunities to test our strengths and abilities in many areas of life. We get to do many, many repetitions of a certain aspect of life. Sometimes we succeed and sometimes we fail but both these times we gain something, which makes us stronger.

A lot of beginning Yoga practitioners have told me that the first change they notice in themselves is that they are becoming more cheerful. We know that cheerfulness is an internal state, starting inside and going outward. When it touches someone, that cheerfulness spreads to the other person. A cheerful person receives a cheerful response most of the time. This is how optimism, creativity, love, and happiness are spread. So, how does the cheerfulness or joyfulness come to the surface? Since it comes to the surface, it implies that it existed there in the first place. It was lying there deep beneath the layers of some other attitudes, some other beliefs and ideas that we held for years. Yoga practice removes the unnecessary layers and frees the mind; and the free mind gets the ability to express love, joy, kindness, and creativity.

Two things we need to recognize are that when we undertake something new, there is some effort involved and it cannot be perfected overnight. We need to commit ourselves over time to get lasting results. Positive results are definitely there. During our journey of Yoga practice, we see the results along the way. We experience some shift in our frame of reference. It is like viewing things from a new vantage point. This shift can have a profound impact on our daily life. The path of evolution is never linear. It is not going straight from point A to point B. It is the path of being open to newness of life and experiencing new discoveries. The new discoveries happen spontaneously when we are in the flow of life. The power of the supercomputer, that is your mind, is amazing and your life is your adventure of many discoveries!

Each of us is born to have a higher purpose in life. We live in a state of "thinking, feeling, and actions" mode, but when we go beyond this mode in deep meditation, we become aware of our higher self. The reverence for all life forms becomes natural as we evolve. We feel the living spirit in all things and that is real awakening. The flow of our breath connects us with all life since all life forms use the same air we breathe in. What a vast resource we all share. As we connect to more beings, we automatically expand in awareness. The thoughts behind the questions, like, "What's the purpose of my life?", "Why am I here?", "Who am I?" will also expand. You will be content with the flow of life. That reward in itself is amazing! Evolution is a win-win aspect of life. Every event brings good to you or it brings something up you need to look at, in order to change you for the better. It is either a gain or a correction, which is also a gain.

Most importantly, you will feel and see the energy that is inside you by practicing Yoga. My sincere hope for you is that you experience that energy and the awareness that comes with it. May your journey of Yoga be filled with new discoveries!

Thank you for your interest in this book, and for reading it. I hope you found it useful and informative. I am certain that you will reap the rewards of your Yoga practice.

I would love to hear from you! If you have any comments or questions, please email me at meenavad@gmail.com

Meena Vad

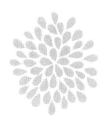

Resources

Chopra, Deepak, *Perfect Health* (New York: Harmony Books, 1991).

Chopra, Deepak, *Ageless Body, Timeless Mind* (New York: Harmony Books, 1993).

Einstein, Albert, *Ideas and Opinions, Essays by Albert Einstein*, Edited by Mein Weltbild, Carl Seelig, and Sonja Bergmann (New York: Wings Books, 1988).

Hewitt James, *The Complete Book of Yoga* (London: Hutchinson Publishing, 1977).

Lad Vasant, *The Complete Book of Ayrvedic Home Remedies* (New York: Three Rivers Press, 1998).

Muktibodhananda, *Hatha Yoga Pradipika* (India: Bihar school of Yoga, 1985).

Ornish, Dean, *Reversing Heart Disease* (New York: Random House Publishing group, 1995).

Peale, Norman Vincent, *Stay Alive All Your Life* (New York: Ballantine Books, 1957).

Peale, Norman Vincent, *The Power of Positive Thinking* (New York: Prentice-Hall Inc. 1958).

Perls, Thomas T., and Silver Margery Hutter, *Living to 100* (New York: Basic Books, 1999).

Rosenthal, Norman, *Transcendence: Healing and Transformation Through Transcendental Meditation* (New York: Penguin Group, 2011)

Sri Swami Satchidananda, *The Yoga Sutras of Patanjali*, 7th ed., trans and commentary (Yogaville, Virginia: Integral Yoga Publications, 1999).

Vivekananda, *The Complete Works of Swami Vivekananda, Volume 1* (Calcutta, India: Advaita Ashram, 1954).

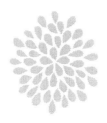

References

1. NCCAM (National Center for Complementary and Alternative Medicine – National Institute of Health) Publication No. D412, May 2008.

2. Dr. Sonia D. Gaur, "Preliminary findings of the Harbor-UCLA Medical Center study" (presented at the American Psychiatric Association's annual meeting in May 2001) and published: *British Medical Journal* 323 (2001):1446-1449; *Annals of Internal Medicine* 135 (2001):262-268

3. "Randomized controlled trial of Yoga and exercise in multiple sclerosis", B.S. Oken, MD; S. Kishiyama, MA; D. Zajdel; D. Bourdette, MD; J. Carlsen, AB; M. Haas, DC, MA; C. Hugos, MS, PT; D.F. Kraemer, PhD; J. Lawrence, BS; M. Mass, MD From the Departments of Neurology (Drs. Oken, Bourdette, and Mass, and S. Kishiyama, D. Zajdel and C. Hugos), Behavioral Neuroscience (Dr. Oken), Rehabilitation (C. Hugos), and Medical Informatics and Clinical Epidemiology (Dr. Kraemer), Oregon Health & Science University, Portland; and Western States Chiropractic College (M. Haas), Portland, OR, 2003.

4. "Long-Term Effects of Stress Reduction on Mortality in Persons > 55 Years of Age With Systemic Hypertension", by Robert H. Schneider, MD, Charles N. Alexander, PhD, Frank Staggers, MD, Maxwell Rainforth, PhD, John W. Salerno, PhD, Arthur Hartz, MD, Stephen Arndt, PhD, Vernon a. Barnes, PhD, and Sanford I. Nidich, EdD (2004), *The American Journal of Cardiology* Vol. 95, (2005).

5. Berk, Lee S. "Neuroendocrine and Stress Hormone Changes During Mirthful Laughter," by Lee Berk, DHSc, Stanley Tan, MD, PhD, William Fry, MD, Barbara Napier, BS, Jerry Lee, PhD, Richard Hubbard, PhD, John Lewis, PhD, William Eby, MD, PhD, *The American Journal of the Medical Sciences* 298, 6 (2009).

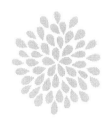

Index

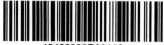
43432385R00116